Exam Preparatory Manual for Nurses Community Health Nursing I

Exam Preparatory Manual for Nurses Community Health Nursing I

As per INC Syllabus

Abha Narwal
MSc Nursing (Community Health Nursing) MSW
Lecturer
Shaheed Baba Deep Singh College of Nursing
Ratia, Fatehabad, Haryana, India

Honey Gangadharan
BSc Nursing MSW PGDHA
Nursing Officer
Dr Ram Manohar Lohia Hospital
New Delhi, India

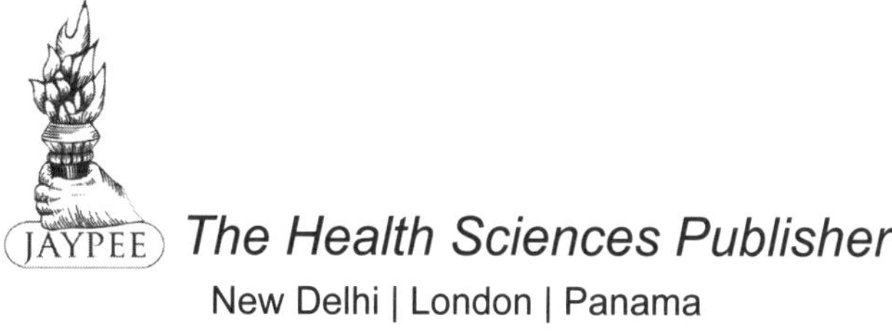

New Delhi | London | Panama

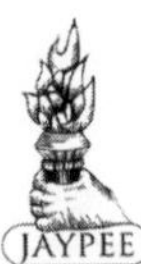

Jaypee Brothers Medical Publishers (P) Ltd

Headquarters

Jaypee Brothers Medical Publishers (P) Ltd.
4838/24, Ansari Road, Daryaganj
New Delhi 110 002, India
Phone: +91-11-43574357
Fax: +91-11-43574314
Email: jaypee@jaypeebrothers.com

Overseas Offices

J.P. Medical Ltd.
83, Victoria Street, London
SW1H 0HW (UK)
Phone: +44-20 3170 8910
Fax: +44-(0)20 3008 6180
Email: info@jpmedpub.com

Jaypee-Highlights Medical Publishers Inc.
City of Knowledge, Bld. 235, 2nd Floor, Clayton
Panama City, Panama
Phone: +1 507-301-0496
Fax: +1 507-301-0499
Email: cservice@jphmedical.com

Jaypee Brothers Medical Publishers (P) Ltd.
Bhotahity, Kathmandu, Nepal
Phone: +977-9741283608
Email: kathmandu@jaypeebrothers.com

Jaypee Brothers Medical Publishers (P) Ltd.
17/1-B, Babar Road, Block-B, Shaymali
Mohammadpur, Dhaka-1207
Bangladesh
Mobile: +08801912003485
Email: jaypeedhaka@gmail.com

Website: www.jaypeebrothers.com
Website: www.jaypeedigital.com

Inquiries for bulk sales may be solicited at: jaypee@jaypeebrothers.com

Exam Preparatory Manual for Nurses Community Health Nursing I

First Edition: **2017**

ISBN 978-93-5270-063-9

Printed at Rajkamal Electric Press, Plot No. 2, Phase-IV, Kundli, Haryana.

Dedicated to
Our Parents and Teachers

Preface

After our last three books caught the attention of the nursing community in a positive way, we were sure that our next project needed to be equally, if not more, critical to nurses. After careful consideration, we decided to take a new approach; one that will help the undergraduates who wish to enter our profession.

The subject of *Community Health Nursing* appears multiple times throughout our study of nursing but still we are devoid of a major reference manual for the same; one that shares the outlook of nursing students. So we decide to bridge that gap with this book—the first part in a series that aims to simplify the subject for easy understanding and quick reproduction during exams.

This book also challenged us in a new way. We had to delve back into our student days and then follow the evolution of the subjects teaching to the latest batches in order to make this book, the easiest to understand while making it a comprehensive text that will not miss any part of significance.

This is our version of a good study-mate for you, that will help you tackle this subject with ease; and we hope you like it.

As always please feel free to reach out to us with your valued suggestions and reviews, which will help us further refine the future editions.

Abha Narwal
Honey Gangadharan

Acknowledgments

Community Health Nursing I has been a real challenge. Not only that it was one of the most important fields in nursing today but also because we wanted it to be a comprehensive guide which covers all academic needs in this relevant field.

For this, our research not only went through the source material at our disposal but also led us to seek recommendations and advice from numerous individuals and groups.

We would like to thank all those who contributed to this project with appropriate and relevant expertise in not just research but also editorial, technical and publishing fields. Without the team effort, this book would not have the quality, expansive coverage and most importantly a student-centric outlook.

We would also like to thank our husbands who have stood by us and enabled us to finish the daunting task and kept encouraging us to further our work.

To the publishers, Jaypee Brothers Medical Publishers (P) Ltd, New Delhi, India who have stuck by us and given us a chance to take a shot at a purely academic project with great belief and support.

Thank you all

Contents

Syllabus → What you have to study → Your syllabus

INC Syllabus

Placement: Second year

Time: Theory-90 hours
Practical-135 hours

Course description: This course is designed for students to appreciate the principles of promotion and maintenance of health

Unit	Time (hrs)	Learning objectives	Content	Teaching learning methods	Assessment method
I	2	• Describe concept and dimensions of health	**Introduction** • Community health nursing • Definition, concept and dimensions of health • Promotion of health • Maintenance of health	• Lecture discussion	• Short answers
II	20	• Describe determinants of health	**Determinants of health** • Eugenics • Environment: – Physical: Air, light, ventilation, water, housing, sanitation; disposal of waste, disposal of dead bodies, Forestation, noise, climate, – Communication: Infrastructure facilities and linkages – Acts regulating the environment: National pollution control board – Bacterial and viral: Agents host carriers and immunity – Arthropods and rodents • Food hygiene: Production, preservation, purchase, preparation, consumption • Acts regulating food hygiene—prevention of food adulteration act, drugs and cosmetic act	• Lecture discussion • Explain using charts, graphs, models, films, slides • Visits to water supply, sewage disposal, milk plants, slaughter house, etc.	• Essay type • Short answers • Objective type

Unit	Time (hrs)	Learning objectives	Content	Teaching learning methods	Assessment method
			• Socio-cultural – Customs, taboos – Marriage system – Family structure – Status of special groups; females, children, elderly, challenged groups and sick persons – Life Style • Hygiene • Physical activity – Recreation and sleep – Sexual life – Spiritual life philosophy – Self reliance – Dietary pattern – Education – Occupation • Financial Management – Income – Budget – Purchasing Power – Security		
III	10	• Describe concept, scope, uses methods and approaches of epidemiology	**Epidemiology** • Definition, concept, aims, scope, uses and terminology used in epidemiology • Dynamics of disease transmission: epidemiological triad • Morbidity and mortality: measurements • Levels of prevention • Methods of epidemiology of – Descriptive – Analytical: Epidemic investigation – Experimental	• Lecture discussion • Explain using charts, graphs, models, films, slides	• Essay type • Short answers
IV	25	• Describe epidemiology and nursing management of common communicable disease	**Epidemiology and nursing management of common communicable diseases** • Respiratory infections – Small pox – Chicken pox	• Lecture discussion • Explain using charts, graphs, models, films, slides • Seminar	• Essay type • Short answers • Objective type

Unit	Time (hrs)	Learning objectives	Content	Teaching learning methods	Assessment method
			– Measles – Influenza – Rubella – ARIs and Pneumonia – Mumps – Diphtheria – Whooping cough – Meningococcal meningitis – Tuberculosis – SARS • Intestinal Infections – Poliomyelitis – Viral Hepatitis – Cholera – Diarrheal Diseases – Typhoid Fever – Food poisoning – Amebiasis – Hookworm infection – Ascariasis – Dracunculiasis • Arthropod infections – Dengue – Malaria – Filariasis • Zoonoses • Viral – Rabies – Yellow fever – Japanese encephalitis – Kyasnur Forest Disease • Bacterial – Brucellosis – Plague – Human Salmonellosis – Anthrax – Leptospirosis • Rickettsial diseases – Rickettsial Zoonoses – Scrub typhus – Murine typhus – Tick typhus – Q fever • Parasitic zoonoses – Taeniasis – Hydatid disease – Leishmaniasis • Surface infection – Trachoma – Tetanus	• Supervised field practice-health centers, clinics and homes • Group projects/ Health education	

Unit	Time (hrs)	Learning objectives	Content	Teaching learning methods	Assessment method
			– Leprosy – STD and RTI – Yaws – HIV/AIDS Any other		
V	10	• Describe epidemiology and nursing management of common noncomm-unicable diseases	**Epidemiology and nursing management of noncommunicable diseases** • Malnutrition: Under nutrition, over nutrition, nutritional deficiencies • Anemia • Hypertension • Stroke • Rheumatic Heart Diseases • Coronary Heart Disease • Cancer • Diabetes mellitus • Blindness • Accidents • Mental illness • Obesity • Iodine Deficiency • Fluorosis • Epilepsy	• Lecture discussion • Explain using charts, graphs, models, films, slides • Seminar • Supervised field practice—health centers, clinics and homes • Group projects/ Health education	• Essay type • Short answers • Objective type
VI	6	• Describe the concepts and scope of demography • Describe method of data collection analysis and interpretation of demographic data	**Demography** • Definition, concept and scope • Methods of collection, analysis and interpretation of demographic data • Demographic rates and ratios	• Lecture discussion • Community identific-ation survey	• Essay type • Short answers • Objective type • Assess-ment of survey report
VII	17	• Identify the impact of population explosion in India • Describe methods of population control	**Population and its control** • Population explosion and its impact on social, economic development of individual, society and country • Population control: – Overall development: Women empowerment, social, economic	• Lecture discussion • Population survey • Counseling • Demonst-ration • Practice session • Supervised field practice	• Essay type • Short answers • Objective type • Assess-ment of survey report

Unit	Time (hrs)	Learning objectives	Content	Teaching learning methods	Assessment method
			and educational development • Limiting family size: – Promotion of small family norm – Methods; spacing (natural, biological, chemical, mechanical method, etc.) – Terminal: Surgical method Emergency Contraception		

Questions → Learn what you have to study → Your questions

1

Introduction to Community Health

LONG ANSWER QUESTIONS

Q.1. a. Define community health nursing.
b. Discuss principles of community health nursing.
c. Explain qualities of community health nurse.
(2 + 4 + 4 = 10 Marks)

Q.2. a. State the objectives and principles of health education. (7 Marks)
b. Discuss the roles and responsibilities of community health nurse in organizing health education program in a village. (8 Marks)

Q.3. a. Define health.
b. Explain the concept of health.
c. Discuss millennium development goals related to health. (2 + 6 + 7 = 15 Marks)

Q.4. a. Discuss the concept 'Health for All' in detail.
b. Explain indicators for health. (7 + 8 = 15 Marks)

SOLVED QUESTIONS PAPER

Q.1. a. Define community health nursing.
b. Discuss principles of community health nursing.
c. Explain qualities of community health nurse.

(A) COMMUNITY HEALTH NURSING

Community health nursing is the synthesis of nursing and public health practice applied to promote and protect the health of population. According to American Nursing Association, 'Community health nursing is a synthesis of nursing practice and public health practice applied in promoting and preserving the health of populations. The nature of this practice is general and comprehensive. It is not limited to a particular age or diagnostic group. It is continuous and not episodic. The dominant responsibility is to the population as a whole'

Community health nursing involves the identification of high-risk aggregates in the community and the development of appropriate and workable policies and interventions to ensure accessible services for all groups of the population.

(B) PRINCIPLES OF COMMUNITY HEALTH NURSING

Community Health Nursing (CHN) is a vital part of Public Health and there are 12 principles to govern CHN.

1. **The recognized need of individuals, families and communities** provides the basis for CHN practice. Its primary purpose is to further apply public health measures within the framework of the total CHN effort.
2. **Knowledge and understanding of the objectives and policies of the agency facilities goal achievement.** The mission statement commits Community Health Nurses to positively actualize their service to this end.
3. **CHN considers the family as the unit of service.** Its level of functioning is influenced by the degree to which it can deal with its own problems. Therefore the family is an effective and available channel for the most of the CHN efforts.
4. **Respect for the values, customs and beliefs** of the clients contribute to the effectiveness of care to the client. CHN services must be available sustainable and affordable to all regardless of race, creed, color or socioeconomic status.
5. **CHN integrated health education and counseling as vital parts of functions.** These encourage and support community efforts in the discussion of issues to improve the people's health.
6. **Collaborative work relationships with the co-workers and members of the health team facilities accomplishments of goals.** Each member is helped to see how his/her work benefits the whole enterprise.

7. **Periodic and continuing evaluation provides the means for assessing the degree to which CHN goals and objectives are being attained.** Clients are involved in the appraisal of their health program through consultations, observations and accurate recording.
8. **Continuing staff education program quality services to client and are essential to upgrade and maintain sound nursing practices in their setting.** Professional interest and needs of Community Health Nurses are considered in planning staff development programs of the agency.
9. **Utilization of indigenous and existing community resources maximizing the success of the efforts of the community health nurses.** The use of local available ailments. Linkages with existing community resources, both public and private, increase the awareness of what care they need what are entitled.
10. **Active participation of the individual, family and community in planning and making decisions for their health care needs determine to a large extent, the success of the CHN programs.** Organized community groups are encouraged to participate in the activities that will meet community needs and interests.
11. **Supervision of nursing services by qualified CHN personnel provides guidance and direction to the work to be done.** Potentials of employees for effective and efficient work are developed.
12. **Accurate recording and reporting serve as the basis for evaluation of the progress of planned programs and activities and as a guide for the future actions.** Maintenance of accurate records is a vital responsibility of community as these are utilized in studies and researches and as legal documents.

(C) QUALITIES OF COMMUNITY HEALTH NURSE

- Efficient
  - Plans with the people, organizes, conducts, directs health education activities according to the needs of the community.
  - Knowledgeable about everything relevant to his practice; has the necessary skills expected of him.
- Good listener
  - Hears what's being said and what's behind the words
  - Always available for the participant to voice out their sentiments and needs

- Keen observer
  - Keep an eye on the proceedings, process and participants' behavior
- Systematic
  - Knows how to put in sequence or logical order the parts of the session
- Creative/Resourceful
  - Uses available resources
- Analytical/Critical thinker
  - Decides on what has been analyzed
- Tactful
  - Brings about issues in smooth subtle manner
  - Does not embarrass but gives constructive criticisms
- Knowledgeable
  - Able to impart relevant, updated and sufficient input
- Open
  - Invites ideas, suggestions, criticisms
  - Involves people in decision making
  - Accepts need for joint planning and decision relative to health care in a particular situation; not resistant to change
- Sense of humor
  - Knows how to place a touch of humor to keep audience alive
- Change agent
  - Involves participants actively in assuming the responsibility for his own learning
- Coordinator
  - Brings into consonance of harmony the community's health care activities
- Objective
  - Unbiased and fair in decision making
- Flexible
  - Able to cope with different situations.

Q.2. a. State the objectives and principles of health education?
b. Discuss the roles and responsibilities of community health nurse in organizing health education program in a village.

(A) HEALTH EDUCATION

Health education is a profession of educating people about health. Areas within this profession encompass environmental health, physical health, social health, emotional health, intellectual health, and spiritual health.

Following are the objectives of health education

- To cultivate the desirable health practices and health habits
- To develop the health attitudes
- To appreciate the health programs undertaken by the school and community and to improve the school and community and to improve the necessary materials for the execution of that program
- To develop health consciousness in the school and in the community
- To teach pupils the rules for the preservation and development of their physical, mental and emotional health
- To eradicate the diseases through health drive programs
- To combat the superstitions and prejudices in the community
- To provide a healthful environment for physical and mental growth.

Following are the principles of health education

- **Interest:** It is a psychological principle that people are unlikely to listen to those things which are not to their interest.
- **Participation:** It should aim at encouraging people to work actively with health workers and others identifying their own health problems and also in developing solution and plans to work them out.
- **Known:** Start where the people are and with what they understand and then proceed to new knowledge.
- **Comprehension:** In health education, we must know the level of understanding, education and literacy of people to whom the teaching directed.
- **Reinforcement:** Repetition at interval is extremely useful for understanding all the news.
- **Motivation:** Every individual has a fundamental desire to learn. Stimulation or awakening of desire of learning called motivation.
- **Communication:** Health educators must be aware of the various barriers of communication and cultural background of the community.
- **Learning by Doing:** The Chinese proverb 'if I hear, I forget. If I see, I remember. If I do, I know' illustrate the importance of learning by doing.

- **Good human relationship:** Maintaining good human relations is essential component of health education.

(B) ROLES AND RESPONSIBILITIES OF COMMUNITY HEALTH NURSE

Nurses play an important role in promoting public health. Traditionally, the focus of health promotion by nurses has been on disease prevention and changing the behavior of individuals with respect to their health. However, their role as promoters of health is more complex, since they have multidisciplinary knowledge and experience of health promotion in their nursing practice. Important points to remember in organizing health education program:

- **Committee formation:** Gather a group of great people to make up your team. Include people who have shown dedication to the issue of health topics as well as people with lots of contacts and energy.
- **Goal formation:** Schedule regular meetings and set goals early.
- **Select message:** Determine what your message will be and to whom you will be sending the message; suggestion: Everyone on your mailing list, local schools, county departments, community centers, hospitals, and pediatricians.
- **Idea generation:** Brainstorm your ideas—ask the 'Magic Wand Question' (What would you see happening if you had a magic wand and no obstacles?) No ideas are bad ideas.
- **Prioritization:** Prioritize as a group. Set goals and then discuss what steps (objectives) you need to take to accomplish those goals.
- **Become task-centered:** Break down the objectives and decide if an individual can manage it or if a team approach is needed. Then assign the tasks.
- **Create a timeline** and if you have e-mail abilities setup a distribution list to keep everyone updated on the progress.
- **Spread the word:** Send a press release or call members of the media (TV and newspaper reporters and editors).
- **Support** each other by keeping in touch with participants. Encourage them to stay on target with the timeline. If someone is having trouble with a task offer help.
- **Follow-up:** Participate activity, and celebrate it at a follow-up meeting.

The roles and responsibilities of community health nurse in organizing health education program in a village are:

- They act as health care educators, providing vital education about the health care options that are available. By leading education campaigns in their communities and raising awareness among community members regarding health issues, community health nurse encourage community members to take charge of their own health.
- Assessment of health complaints, medication administration, and care for people with special health care needs.
- Mandated health screening programs, verification of immunizations, and infectious disease reporting.
- Identification and management of chronic health care needs that affect educational achievement.
- Establish a participatory team in a rural county composed of youth, parents, and trusted community leaders.
- Conduct a community and environmental assessment with the team to identify ecological, cultural, and contextual factors influencing substance-free and substance-using adolescent lifestyles.
- Evaluate the effectiveness of prevention programs in light of the community's ecological, cultural, and contextual dimensions, health attitudes and behaviors, and on that basis develop a tobacco, alcohol, and drug use preventive intervention for this rural tobacco-producing community.

Q.3. a. Define health.
b. Explain the concept of health.
c. Discuss millennium development goals related to health.

(A) HEALTH

Health is a state of complete physical, mental and social well-being and not merely an absence of disease or infirmity—WHO, 1948.

Operational definition of Health by WHO—a condition or quality of the human organism expressing the adequate functioning of the organism in given conditions, genetic or environmental.

Health is the soundness of the body, mind or spirit, especially the state of being free from diseases or pain—Bevster.

(B) CONCEPT OF HEALTH

- **Biomedical concept:** Biomedical concept is based on the principle of germs. According to this concept, human body is a machine; disease is the failure of machine and the treatment means the repair of machine. If a human body is free from disease then the individual is considered healthy. This concept has minimized the role of environmental, social, cultural and other factors that influences health.
- **Ecological concept:** This concept is based on the hypothesis that there is a transient balance between the man and his environment. Health is a dynamic equilibrium between man and his environment. Disease is maladjustment of the human organisms to the environment. According to this concept, ill health is related to the imbalance between the man and his environment. This concept supports the need for clean air, safe water, ozone layer, etc. to protect from exposure to unhealthy factors.
- **Psychosocial concept:** Health is not only a biomedical concept; as it is also influenced by social, psychological, cultural, political and other factors.
- **Holistic concept:** This concept involves biomedical, ecological, psychosocial factors together. It is defined as a multidimensional process involving the well-being of the whole person in the context of his environment.
- **Concept of well-being:** It involves two components; one is objective component other is subjective.
  - **Objective component:**
    - **Standard of living:** Refers to the usual scale of our expenditure, the goods we consume and the service we enjoy. It includes the level of education, employment status, food, dress, house, amusement and comforts of modern living. WHO: 'Income and occupation, standard of housing, sanitation and nutrition, the level of provision of health, educational, recreational and other services.
    - **Level of living:** Mainly used in US. Covers 9 components:
      - Health
      - Food consumption

  - Education
  - Occupation and working condition
  - Housing
  - Social security
  - Clothing
  - Recreation and leisure
  - Human right.
- **Subjective component:**
  - **Quality of Life:** The condition of life resulting from the combination of the effects of the complete range of factors such as those determining health, happiness (including comfort in the physical environment and the satisfying occupation), education, social and intellectual attainments, freedom of action, justice and freedom of expression. A composite measure of physical, mental and social well-being as perceived by each individual or group of individuals.

(C) MILLENNIUM DEVELOPMENT GOALS RELATED TO HEALTH

The Millennium Development Goals (MDGs) were the eight international development goals for the year 2015 that had been established following the Millennium Summit of the United Nations in 2000. Following the adoption of the United Nations Millennium Declaration, all 189 United Nations member states at that time, and at least 22 international organizations, committed to help, achieve the following Millennium Development Goals by 2015:

1. To eradicate extreme poverty and hunger
2. To achieve universal primary education
3. To promote gender equality and empower women
4. To reduce child mortality
5. To improve maternal health
6. To combat HIV/AIDS, malaria, and other diseases
7. To ensure environmental sustainability
8. To develop a global partnership for development.

Health-related Millennium Development Goals and Targets

Goal 1: Eradicate poverty and hunger

Target 1.C: Halve, between 1990 and 2015, the proportion of people who suffer from hunger.

Goal 4: Reduce child mortality
Target 4.A: Reduce by two-thirds, between 1990 and 2015, the under-five mortality rate.

Goal 5: Improve maternal health
Target 5.A: Reduce by three quarters, between 1990 and 2015, the maternal mortality ratio.
Target 5.B: Achieve, by 2015, universal access to reproductive health.

Goal 6: Combat HIV/AIDS, malaria and other diseases
Target 6.A: Have halted by 2015 and begun to reverse the spread of HIV/AIDS.
Target 6.B: Achieve, by 2010, universal access to treatment for HIV/AIDS for all those who need it.
Target 6.C: Have halted by 2015 and begun to reverse the incidence of malaria and other major diseases.

Goal 7: Ensure environmental sustainability
Target 7.C: Halve, by 2015, the proportion of people without sustainable access to safe drinking water and basic sanitation.

Goal 8: Develop a global partnership for development
Target 8.E: In cooperation with pharmaceutical companies, provide access to affordable essential drugs in developing countries.

Q.4. a. Discuss the concept 'Health for All' in detail.
b. Explain indicators for health.

(A) HEALTH FOR ALL

In 1977, the World Health Assembly decided that the main social target of governments and of WHO should be the attainment by all the people of the word by the year 2000 of a level of health that would permit them to lead a socially and economically productive life. In other worlds, as a minimum, all people in all countries should have at least such a level of health that they are capable of working productively and of participating actively in the social life of the community in which they live. The third evaluation of progress in implementing the Global Strategy for Health for All by the year 2000 (carried out in 1997) has shown significant improvements worldwide both in health status and in access to health care.

Increasing numbers of Member States are carrying out monitoring and evaluation of their health-for-all strategies at specified intervals; for the first evaluation in 1985, 147 out of 166 Member States reported, at least with respect to the global indicators. In 1997, 158 out of 191 Member States did so, although some indicators were more widely covered than others, e.g. 90% of countries reported on immunization, but only 30% on access to local health services.

Definition: Halfdan Mahler, Director General (1973–1983) of the WHO, defined Health for All in 1981, as follows:

Health for All means that health is to be brought within reach of everyone in a given country. And by 'health' is meant a personal state of well-being, not just the availability of health services—a state of health that enables a person to lead a socially and economically productive life. Health for All implies the removal of the obstacles to health—that is to say, the elimination of malnutrition, ignorance, contaminated drinking water and unhygienic housing—quite as much as it does the solution of purely medical problems such as a lack of doctors, hospital beds, drugs and vaccines.

- Health for All means that health should be regarded as an objective of economic development and not merely as one of the means of attaining it.
- Health for All demands, ultimately, literacy for all. Until this becomes reality, it demands at least the beginning of an understanding of what health means for every individual.
- Health for All depends on continued progress in medical care and public health. The health services must be accessible to all through primary health care, in which basic medical help is available in every village, backed up by referral services to more specialized care. Immunization must similarly achieve universal coverage.
- Health for All is thus a holistic concept calling for efforts in agriculture, industry, education, housing, and communications, just as much as in medicine and public health. Medical care alone cannot bring health to in hovels. Health for such people requires a whole new way of life and fresh opportunities to provide themselves with a higher standard of living.

The adoption of Health for All by government, implies a commitment to promote the advancement of all citizens on a broad front of development and a resolution to encourage the individual citizen to achieve a higher quality of life.

The rate of progress will depend on the political will. The World Health Assembly believes that, given a high degree of determination, Health for All could be attained by the year 2000. That target date is a challenge to all WHO's Member States.

The basis of the Health for All strategy is primary health care.

(B) INDICATORS OF HEALTH

A health indicator is a single measure that is reported on regularly and that provides relevant and actionable information about population health and/or health system performance and characteristics. An indicator can provide comparable information, as well as track progress and performance over time. Health indicators support provinces/territories, regional health authorities and facilities as they monitor the health of their populations and track how well their local health systems function.

A health indicator which will be used internationally to describe global health should have the following characteristics:

- It should be valid; they should actually measure what they are supposed to measure
- It should be specific; they should reflect changes only in the situation concerned.
- It should be defined in such a way that it can be measured uniformly internationally.
- It should be reliable; as it yields the same result if measured by different people in same circumstances.
- The indicator must be data which can feasibly be collected.
- The analysis of the data must result in a recommendation on which people can make changes to improve health.

The health indicators include:

- Mortality indicators
  - Crude death rate
  - Life expectancy
  - Infant mortality rate
  - Maternal mortality rate
  - Proportional mortality rate
- Morbidity indicators
  - Prevalence
  - Incidence
  - Others

- Health status
  - Low birth weight
  - Obesity
  - Arthritis
  - Diabetes
  - Asthma
  - High blood pressure
  - Cancer incidence
  - Chronic pain
- Disability indicators
  - Disability adjusted life years (DALY)
  - Others: Activities of daily living (ADL), Musculoskeletal disability (MSD) score, etc.
- Nutritional indicators
  - Proportion of low birth weight
  - Prevalence of anemia
  - Proportion of overweight individuals
  - Nutritional intake assessments
- Social and mental health indicators
  - Alcohol related indicators
  - Injury rates
- Health system indicators
  - Health care delivery related
  - Health policy indicators.

SHORT NOTES

(5 Marks)

Q.1. Dimensions of health

Q.2. Modes of intervention

Q.3. Eugenics

Q.4. Ergonomics

Q.5. Spectrum of health

Q.6. Levels of prevention:

Q.7. Health illness continuum

Q.8. Difference between institutional and community health nursing

Q.9. Determinants of health

SOLVED QUESTIONS PAPER

1. DIMENSIONS OF HEALTH

Health: Health is a state of complete physical, mental and social well-being and not merely the absence of disease or infirmity. —WHO, 1948.

Dimensions of health: The term wellness can refer to a variety of conditions within the body. While many people associate their wellness to their physical health, it can also be used to describe your environmental, mental, intellectual, occupational, emotional or spiritual well-being. These different dimensions of health will interact together to help determine your full quality of life.

Seven dimensions of health are:

1. **Physical:** Physical dimension of health denotes the perfect functioning of the body. It can refer to any of the aspects that are needed to keep your body in top condition. Consuming a healthy diet and getting an adequate amount of exercise to build cardiovascular health, endurance or flexibility are essential to this goal. Signs of good physical health are a clear skin, good complexion, a sweat breath, good appetite, bright eyes, lustrous hair, regular activity of bowel and bladder, etc.
2. **Mental:** Finding a way to engage in creative and stimulating activities that allow you to share your gifts and expand your knowledge is essential to your overall health. This will allow you to find a path to explore your creativity, problem solving skills and ways to learn more about your personal interests and the world around you. Keeping up with current events and finding new ideas to strike your intellectual curiosity will allow you to continue to grow over time. Attributes of a mentally healthy individual are:
   - They feel good about themselves.
   - They do not become overwhelmed by emotions, such as fear, anger, love, jealousy, guilt, or anxiety.
   - They have lasting and satisfying personal relationships.
   - They feel comfortable with other people.
   - They can laugh at themselves and with others.
   - They have respect for themselves and for others even if there are differences.
   - They are able to accept life's disappointments.

- They can meet life's demands and handle their problems when they arise.
- They make their own decisions.
- They shape their environment whenever possible and adjust to it when necessary.

3. **Emotional:** Emotional wellness focuses on ensuring that you are attentive to your feelings, thoughts and behavior. This includes both positive and negative reactions, though overall you should:

- Seek an optimistic approach to life, enjoying life in spite of occasional disappointments.
- Adjust to change and express your emotions appropriately.
- Express your feelings freely while managing your feelings, allowing yourself to cope with stress in a way that is healthy.

4. **Spiritual:** Spiritual wellness involves discovering a set of beliefs and values that brings purpose to your life. While different groups and individuals have a variety of beliefs regarding spiritualism but the general search for meaning for our existence is considered essential to creating harmony with yourself and others regardless of the path to spirituality you choose to follow.
5. **Social:** Social wellness refers to your ability to interact with people, respect yourself and others, develop meaningful relationships and develop quality communication skills. This allows you to establish a support system of family and friends.
6. **Occupational:** The ability to find peace between your leisure time and work time while managing stress from your relationships with co-workers effectively is essential to occupational health. Your work takes up a great deal of your time so it is important to find something that you love to do and gives you a sense of purpose.
7. **Environmental:** The environment can have a significant impact on our feelings about overall health. For developing environmental wellness, you should:

- Live in harmony with your environment.
- Take action to protect this environment from harm.
- Minimize behavior that could impact your environment while protecting yourself from environmental hazards.
- Realize the effects of your daily habits on the world around you.
- Live a life that is accountable to your short- and long-term environmental needs.
- Bring awareness of the Earth's limits and resource to others.

A few other dimensions have also been suggested such as philosophical dimension, cultural dimension, socioeconomical dimension, educational dimension, nutritional dimension, etc.

2. MODES OF INTERVENTION

In medicine, an intervention is usually undertaken to help treat or cure a condition. It is an attempt to interrupt the usual sequence in the development of disease. There are 5 modes of interventions;

1. Health promotion: It is aimed at improving the general health and quality of life of individuals and the community. It involves a comprehensive approach towards changes in lifestyle and human behavior.

There are four areas of health promotion:

i. **Health education:** A large number of diseases can be prevented if people are adequately explained about it by using little or no medical treatment. Knowledge about health legislation, family planning, marriage counseling, sex education, improving personal hygiene, etc.
ii. **Environment modifications:** Includes provision of safe water, good housing installation of sanitary latrines, keeping environment rodents free, etc.
iii. **Nutritional interventions:** Includes food fortification, nutritional improvement of vulnerable groups, prevention of food adulteration, nutrition education, etc.
iv. **Lifestyle and behavioral changes:** Includes limiting the use of tobacco, alcohol and drugs, keeping oneself physically fit, etc.

2. Specific protection: It refers to specific measures taken to prevent the occurrence of disease. These measures include:

- Immunization
- Chemoprophylaxis
- Use of specific nutrients
- Protection of occupational hazards by using gloves, goggles, shields, etc.
- Protection against accidents
- Avoidance of allergy
- Protection from cancer producing agents
- Avoidance of allergens.

3. Early diagnosis and treatment: It is the main intervention in disease control. It is like stamping out the 'spark' rather than calling the fire brigade to put out the fire. If the disease is diagnosed and treated earlier, it will prevent complications and also secondary cases in the community.

Methods employed for early diagnosis are:

- Individual and mass case finding
- Screening and surveys
- Periodic examination
- Special examination of people at risk.

Treatment depends on the nature of the disease and its condition.

4. Disability limitation: It is the intervention taken in the stage of late pathogenesis. Disability limitation prevents complications and also prevents or postpones death. The major causes of disability are communicable diseases, malnutrition, lack of parental care and accidents.

Disability can be prevented by:

- Reducing the occurrence of impairment, e.g. polio immunization
- Appropriate treatment, e.g. treatment of thromboangiitis obliterans (TAO) can prevent amputation
- Preventing the disability to produce handicap, e.g. preventing loss of employment in case of loss of limb.

5. Rehabilitation: It is the combined and coordinated use of medical, social, educational and vocational measures for training and retraining the individual to the highest possible level of functional ability.

The different types of rehabilitation are:

- **Medical rehabilitation:** It is restoration of function.
- **Vocational rehabilitation:** It is restoration of the capacity to earn livelihood.
- **Social rehabilitation:** It is the restoration of family and social relationships.
- **Psychological rehabilitation:** It is restoration of personal dignity and confidence.

Examples of rehabilitation are:

- Provision of aids to the crippled
- Establishment of blind schools
- Reconstructive surgery for leprosy
- Physiotherapy and exercise in polio cases
- Change to a suitable occupation
- Reassurance and socially accepting leprosy patients
- Modification of life in general and especially in cardiac patients.

3. EUGENICS

Eugenics is a set of beliefs and practices that aims at improving the genetic quality of the human population. Eugenics is the science of using controlled, selective breeding to improve hereditary qualities of the human race. Francis Galton is the father of Eugenics. He believed that biology is not only responsible for physical characteristics but mental as well.

Types: It is a social philosophy advocating the improvement of human genetic traits through the promotion of higher rates of sexual reproduction for people with desired traits (positive eugenics), or reduced rates of sexual reproduction and sterilization of people with less-desired or undesired traits (negative eugenics), or both.

Alternatively, gene selection rather than 'people selection' has recently been made possible through advances in gene editing (e.g. CRISPR). The exact definition of eugenics has been a matter of debate since the term was coined. The definition of it as a 'social philosophy'—that is, a philosophy with implications for social order—is not universally accepted, and was taken from Frederick Osborn's 1937 journal article 'Development of a Eugenic Philosophy'.

Methods of Eugenics

- **Mandatory eugenics:** Government mandated
- **Promotional voluntary eugenics:** Suggested to the general population
- **Private eugenics:** Voluntary participation

While eugenic principles have been practiced as far back in world history as Ancient Greece, the modern history of eugenics began in the early 20th century when a popular eugenics movement emerged in the United Kingdom and spread to many countries, including the United States and most European countries.

In this period, eugenic ideas were espoused across the political spectrum. Consequently, many countries adopted eugenic policies meant to improve the genetic stock of their countries. Such programs often included both positive measures, such as encouraging individuals deemed particularly fit to reproduce, and negative measures such as marriage prohibitions and forced sterilization of people deemed unfit for reproduction. People deemed unfit to reproduce often included people with mental or physical disabilities, people who scored in the low ranges of different IQ tests, criminals and deviants, and members of disfavored minority groups.

The eugenics movement became negatively associated with Nazi Germany and the Holocaust when many of the defendants at the Nuremberg trials attempted to justify their human rights abuses by claiming there was little difference between the Nazi eugenics programs and the US eugenics programs. In the decades following World War II, with the institution of human rights, many countries gradually abandoned eugenics policies, although some Western countries, among them the United States, continued to carry out forced sterilizations.

4. ERGONOMICS

Ergonomics is the scientific study of people at work. The goal of ergonomics is to reduce stress and eliminate injuries and disorders associated with the overuse of muscles, bad posture, and repeated tasks. This is accomplished by designing tasks, work spaces, controls, displays, tools, lighting, and equipment to fit the employee's physical capabilities and limitations.

Domains of Specialization: Derived from the Greek ergon (work) and nomos (laws) to denote the science of work, ergonomics is a systems-oriented discipline which now extends across all aspects of human activity. Practicing ergonomists must have a broad understanding of the full scope of the discipline.

- **Physical Ergonomics:** Physical ergonomics is concerned with human anatomical, anthropometric, physiological and biomechanical characteristics as they relate to physical activity. (Relevant topics include working postures, materials handling, repetitive movements, work related musculoskeletal disorders, workplace layout, safety and health.)
- **Cognitive Ergonomics:** Cognitive ergonomics is concerned with mental processes, such as perception, memory, reasoning, and motor response, as they affect interactions among humans and other elements of a system. (Relevant topics include mental workload, decision-making, skilled performance, human-computer interaction, human reliability, work stress and training as these may relate to human-system design.)
- **Organizational Ergonomics:** Organizational ergonomics is concerned with the optimization of sociotechnical systems, including their organizational structures, policies, and

processes. (Relevant topics include communication, crew resource management, work design, design of working times, teamwork, participatory design, community ergonomics, cooperative work, new work paradigms, virtual organizations, telework, and quality management.)

Methods: Until recently, methods used to evaluate human factors and ergonomics ranged from simple questionnaires to more complex and expensive usability labs. Some of the more common human factor and ergonomics (HF & E) methods are listed below:

- **Ethnographic analysis:** It is a qualitative and observational method that focuses on 'real-world' experience and pressures, and the usage of technology or environments in the workplace.
- **Focus Groups** are another form of qualitative research in which one individual will facilitate discussion and elicit opinions about the technology or process under investigation. This can be on a one to one interview basis, or in a group session.
- **Iterative design:** Also known as prototyping, the iterative design process seeks to involve users at several stages of design, in order to correct problems as they emerge.
- **Meta-analysis:** A supplementary technique used to examine a wide body of already existing data or literature in order to derive trends or form hypotheses in order to aid design decisions.
- **Subjects-in-tandem:** Two subjects are asked to work concurrently on a series of tasks while vocalizing their analytical observations.
- **Surveys and Questionnaires**
- **Task analysis:** A process with roots in activity theory, task analysis is a way of systematically describing human interaction with a system or process to understand how to match the demands of the system or process to human capabilities.
- **Methods Analysis** is the process of studying the tasks a worker completes using a step-by-step investigation. Each task is broken down into smaller steps until each motion the worker performs is described. Doing so enables you to see exactly where repetitive or straining tasks occur.
- **Time studies** determine the time required for a worker to complete each task. Time studies are often used to analyze cyclical jobs. They are considered 'event based' studies because time measurements are triggered by the occurrence of predetermined events.

- **Work sampling** is a method in which the job is sampled at random intervals to determine the proportion of total time spent on a particular task. It provides insight into how often workers are performing tasks which might cause strain on their bodies.
- **Macroergonomic Analysis of Structure (MAS):** This method analyzes the structure of work systems according to their compatibility with unique sociotechnical aspects.
- **Macroergonomic Analysis and Design (MEAD):** This method assesses work-system processes by using a ten-step process.
- **Virtual Manufacturing and Response Surface Methodology (VMRSM):** This method uses computerized tools and statistical analysis for workstation design.

Limitations of these methods:

- Usually take more time and resources than other methods.
- Very high effort in planning, recruiting, and executing than other methods
- Much longer study periods and therefore requires much goodwill among the participants
- Studies are longitudinal in nature, therefore, attrition can become a problem.

5. SPECTRUM OF HEALTH

Spectrum of health emphasizes that health of an individual is a dynamic phenomenon and a process of continuous change subject to repeated and fine variations. Transition from optimum health to ill health is often gradual and where one state ends and other begins is a matter of judgment.

Spectrum refers to the image of the band of colors formed by a ray of light that has passed through a prism. As it is difficult to distinguish the beginning, end or boundaries of color; likewise it is also difficult to differentiate spectrum of health. To describe health as the absence of disease is inadequate and unsatisfying. We have defined diseases for the last four hundred years or so according to the presence of certain lesions, or the presence of 'abnormal' readings measured by instruments of investigation. Illness is a related, but different, term from disease. It is used mainly to refer to the experience of being unwell, incorporating our concept of disease, but actually describing the subjective experience of a person.

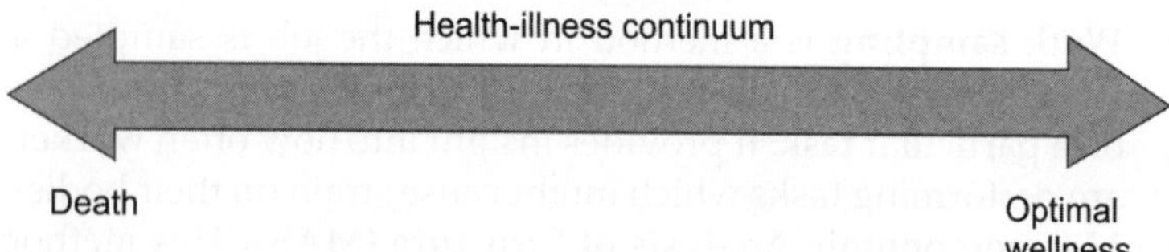

Current views of health and illness recognize health as more than the absence of disease. Realizing that humans are dynamic beings whose state of health can change from day to day or even from hour to hour. Medical researchers suggest that it is better to think of each person as being located on a continuous scale (continuum) ranging from death to a state of optimal functioning, i.e. positive health. High-level wellness is described as a dynamic process in which the individual is actively engaged in moving towards fulfillment of his or her potential.

- Health and disease lie along a continuum, and there is no single cut off point.
- The lowest point on the health-disease spectrum is death and the highest point corresponds to the WHO definition of positive health.
- Health fluctuates within a range of optimal well-being to various levels of dysfunction, including the state of total dysfunction, namely death.
- The transition from optimum health to ill health of often gradual and where one ends other state begins.
- The spectrum concept of health emphasizes that the health of an individual is not static; is a dynamic phenomenon and a process of continuous change, subject to frequent subtle variations. What is considered maximum may be considered minimum tomorrow.
- A person may function at maximum levels of health today and may be minimum tomorrow.
- It implies that health is a state not to be attained once and for all, but ever to be renewed. There are degrees or 'levels of health' as there are severity of illnesses.

6. LEVELS OF PREVENTION

There are four levels of prevention.

1. Primordial prevention: This is a prevention of emergence or development of risk factors in a population group. Special attention is given to preventing chronic diseases. Main intervention is health

Spectrum of health

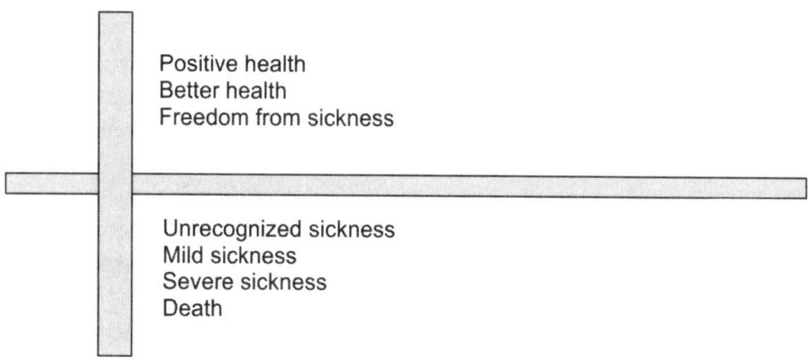

education. In this, efforts are directed towards discouraging children from adopting harmful styles.

2. Primary prevention: In this, action is taken before the onset of disease. Primary preventive measures apply before a disease manifests with signs and symptoms.

- **Health promotion:** For example, health education, environment modification, nutritional intervention, behavior change, etc.
- **Specific protection:** For example, immunization, use of specific nutrients, chemoprophylaxis, protection against accident, carcinogens, etc.

3. Secondary prevention: This is aimed at patients with an existing pathology to reduce the risk of recurrence or progression. Early diagnosis and treatment are the intervention for secondary prevention. For example, all the screening test, Aspirin in arterial disease. Secondary prevention increases awareness of Breast self-examination, testicular self-examination, mammography, PAP smear, BP screening, etc.

4. Tertiary prevention: It is aimed at avoiding further deterioration of an already existing situation. All measures to reduce or limit disability and impairment minimize suffering caused by disease process. Interventions include:

- Disability limitation
- **Rehabilitation:** Rehabilitation is restoration of an individual or a part of normal or near normal functions after disability, disease. It can be:
  - **Medical rehabilitation:** Restoration of function.
  - **Vocational rehabilitation:** Restoration of the capacity to earn a livelihood.

- **Social rehabilitation:** Restoration of family and social relation.
- **Psychological rehabilitation:** Restoration of personal dignity and confidence.

7. HEALTH ILLNESS CONTINUUM

Health and disease lie along a continuum and there is no single cut-off point. The lowest point on the health and disease spectrum is death and highest point corresponds to the WHO definition of positive health. It is thus obvious that health fluctuates within a range of optimum well-being to various levels of dysfunction, namely the death. The transition from optimum health to ill health is often gradual, and where state ends and the other begin is a matter of judgment.

So the spectral concept of health of an individual is not static. It is a dynamic phenomenon and a process of continuous change, subject to frequent stable variations. What considering maximum health is today may be minimum tomorrow

That is a person may function at maximum level of health today and diminished level of health tomorrow. It implies that health is a state not to be attained once and for all, but ever to be renewed. There are degrees or 'levels of health 'as there are degrees or severity of illness. As long as we are alive there is some degree of health in us.

Health illness continuum model: Health always involves a continuum a range of degree from optimal health at one end to death or total disability at the other. The health of an individual moves back and forth along this continuum throughout life according to health and illness continuum model. Health is a dynamic state fluctuates as a person adapts to change in the internal and external environment to maintain a state of total well-being.

High-level of wellness and severe illness are at opposite ends of the continuum. According the Neumann's 1990 health on a continuum is the degree of clients wellness that exist at any point in time running from an optimal wellness condition, with available energy at its maximum to death which represents total energy depletion. Risk factors are important in identifying level of health. They include genetic and physiological variables such as age, lifestyle, and environment.

- According to this model, health is a dynamic state that fluctuates as a person adapts to changes in the internal or external environments to maintain a state of well-being.

- Illness is a process in which the functioning of a client is diminished or impaired when compared with his/ her previous condition.
- In this model, high-level wellness and severe illness are at opposite ends of the continuum.

Risk factors, including genetic and physiological, environmental age, and lifestyle, are at the center of the model.

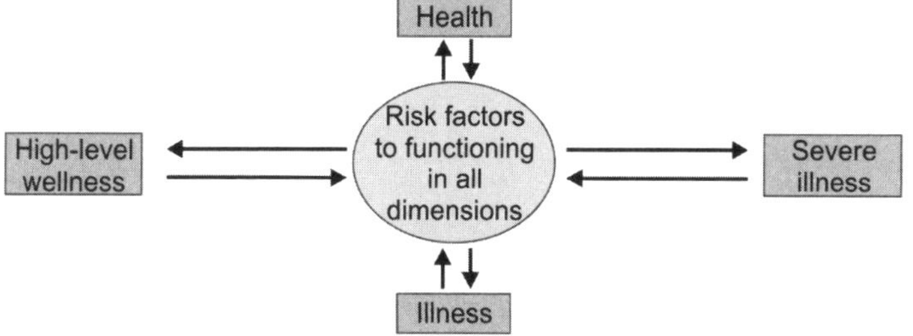

8. DIFFERENCE BETWEEN INSTITUTIONAL AND COMMUNITY HEALTH NURSING

The difference between institutional and community health nursing is mentioned below:

S.No.	Institutional nursing	Community health nursing
1	Deliver health services to the patient admitted in the hospital	Deliver health services to the individual, families and communities
2	The goal of the institutional nurse is to help the patient get well enough to go home from the hospital	The goal of the community health nurse is to keep the patient at home and prevent hospitalization or long-term care in an institution
3	Patient comes to the hospital himself. No motivation required.	Patient is to be motivated by the community nurse for diagnosis, treatment and follow-up treatment in their home or work of place
4	Work place is mainly hospitals, home, slums, health center, etc.	Work place is mostly the community, e.g. clinic, school, health center, etc.
5	Staff usually have expertise in one branch	For CH nurse, it is essential to have knowledge of all branches of medical science

Contd..

Contd..

S.No.	Institutional nursing	Community health nursing
6	Records of patient are generally stored by the medical record department	Storage and maintenance of medical records of patient is done by community nurse
7	They are more concerned with the causes and diagnosis of disease and treatment of the patient	It is concerned with all aspects of health, i.e. diagnosis, treatment, health promotion, rehabilitation, etc.
8	Specialist doctors or senior colleagues are available to decide about treatment	Mostly decision is taken by community nurse regarding decision related to the treatment of patient
9	Interpersonal relation is maintained with the patient	Here, along with interpersonal public relation is also maintained
10	Nurses at hospitals deal with illnesses usually after they have progressed	Community nursing aims to lower the risk of patients needed hospital treatments

9. DETERMINANTS OF HEALTH

The range of personal, social, economic, and environmental factors that influence health status are known as determinants of health.

Determinants of health fall under several broad categories:
The context of people's lives determines their health, and so blaming individuals for having poor health or crediting them for good health is inappropriate. Individuals are unlikely to be able to directly control many of the determinants of health. These determinants—or things that make people healthy or not—include the above factors, and many others:

- **Income and social status:** Higher income and social status are linked to better health. The greater the gap between the richest and poorest people, the greater the differences in health.
- **Education:** Low education levels are linked with poor health, more stress and lower self-confidence.
- **Physical environment:** Safe water and clean air, healthy workplaces, safe houses, communities and roads all contribute to good health. Employment and working conditions—people in employment are healthier, particularly those who have more control over their working conditions.
- **Social support networks:** Greater support from families, friends and communities is linked to better health. Culture—customs and traditions, and the beliefs of the family and community all affect health.

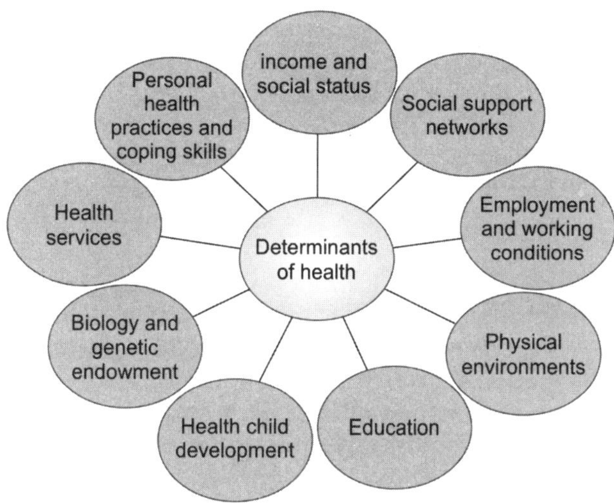

- **Genetics:** Inheritance plays a part in determining lifespan, healthiness and the likelihood of developing certain illnesses. Personal behavior and coping skills—balanced eating, keeping active, smoking, drinking, and how we deal with life's stresses and challenges all affect health.
- **Health services:** Access and use of services that prevent and treat disease influences health.
- **Gender:** Men and women suffer from different types of diseases at different ages.

VERY SHORT ANSWER QUESTIONS

(2 Marks)

Q.1. What is the basic unit of service in community health nursing?

Ans. Community Health Nursing considers the family as the unit of service. Its level of functioning is influenced by the degree to which it can deal with its own problems. Therefore the family is an effective and available channel for the most of its efforts.

Q.2. Concept of well-being.

Ans. Well-being is a general term for the condition of an individual or group, for example their social, economic, psychological, spiritual or medical state; a high-level of well-being means in some sense the individual or group's condition is positive, while low well-being is associated with negative happenings. Well-being has three components:

1. **Standard of living:** Refers to the usual scale of our expenditure, the goods we consume and the service we enjoy. It includes the level of education, employment status, food, dress, house, amusement and comforts of modern living.
2. **Level of living:** It includes health, food consumption, education, occupation and working condition, housing, social security, clothing, human right, recreation and leisure.
3. **Quality of life:** The condition of life resulting from the combination of the effects of the complete range of factors such as those determining health, happiness (including comfort in the physical environment and the satisfying occupation), education, social and intellectual attainments, freedom of action, justice and freedom of expression.

Q.3. Define death rate.

Ans. The Death Rate is defined as the number of deaths per 1000 estimated midyear population in one year. It is given by formula.

$$\text{Death rate} = \frac{\text{Number of death during year}}{\text{Estimated midyear population}} \times 1000$$

Q.4. Define epidemic and give one example.

Ans. An epidemic is the rapid spread of infectious disease to a large number of people in a given population within a short period of time, usually two weeks or less. For example, meningococcal infections, an attack rate in excess of 15 cases per 100,000 people for two consecutive weeks is considered an epidemic.

Q5. Explain human development index.

Ans. HDI is an index used to rank countries by level of human development which usually also implies whether a country is developed, developing or underdeveloped.

HDI is defined as a composite index combining indicators representing three dimensions; longevity, knowledge and income. Combines indicators representing three dimensions:

- **Longevity:** Life expectancy at birth
- **Knowledge:** Adult literacy rate and mean year of schooling.
- **Income:** Real GDP per capita in purchasing power parity (PPP) in US dollars

$$\text{Index} = \frac{\text{(Actual Value)} - \text{(Minimum Value)}}{\text{(Maximum Value)} - \text{(Minimum Value)}}$$

Q.6 Explain disease cycle.

Ans. Disease cycle has six stages:

- **Incubation period:** Time interval between entry of infective organism in body of host and appearance of first symptom or sign.
- **Prodrome:** Period immediately following onset characterized by vague or non-specific symptoms. It is difficult to diagnose at this stage.
- **Fastigium:** It is the period when the disease is at its maximum severity. Stage during which classical signs and symptoms are present.
- **Defervescence:** It is the period when the symptoms of the illness are declining.
- **Convalescence:** Patient recovered from the illness but patient is too exhausted or weak to carry out activities of daily living (ADL).
- **Defection:** It is the period during which the pathogen is killed off or brought to remission.

Q.7 Differentiate between surveillance and monitoring.

S.No.	*Surveillance*	*Monitoring*
1	It is defined as the continuous scrutiny of the factors that determine the occurrence and distribution of diseases and other health related states.	It is defined as the performance and analysis of routine analysis aimed at detecting changes of selected indicators.
2	It is a continuous cycle.	It is one time activity.
3	Feedback is present.	There is no feedback in monitoring.

Q8. Explain herd immunity.

Ans. Level of resistance of a community or a group of people to a particular disease. Herd Immunity is a form of indirect protection from infectious disease that occurs when a large percentage of a population has become immune to an infection, thereby providing a measure of protection for individuals who are not immune. Even individuals not vaccinated (such as newborns and those with chronic illnesses) are offered some protection because the disease has little opportunity to spread within the community. Also known as community immunity.

Q9. Explain notification of disease.

Ans: Notification of disease is the prompt reporting of defined communicable diseases to appropriate health authorities.

Types of disease notification:

- Local notification: Reporting of disease done within limits of local are in respect to disease.
- National notification: Reporting of the disease according to public health importance of disease in that country.
- International notification: Helps in identifying nature and behavior of disease. It is useful in providing data for monitoring of incidence and prevalence of disease on an international level.

Q10. Differentiate between active and passive immunity.

S.no.	Active immunity	Passive immunity
1.	Active immunity is produced due to contact with the pathogen.	Passive immunity is produced due to antibodies obtained from outside.
2.	Immunity is not immediate in active immunity; a time lapse occurs for its development.	In passive immunity, immunity develops immediately.
3.	Protective efficiency is higher in active immunity.	Protective efficiency is less.
4.	In active immunity, cost of immunization is cheaper.	Cost of immunization is expensive.
5.	Antibodies are produced by the body in response to the pathogen or antigen	Antibodies are obtained from outside.
6.	Immunologic memory may result in lifelong immunity.	It lasts for a few days.

Q11. Define Sullivan`s index.

Ans: Sullivan`s Index is also known as disability-free life expectancy (DFLE). It is a method to compute life expectancy free of disability. It is calculated by formula:

Sullivan's Index = Life expectancy – Duration of disability.

- Health expectancy calculated by Sullivan's method is the number of remaining years, at a particular age, that an individual can expect to live in a healthy state.
- It is computed by subtracting the probable duration of bed disability and inability to perform major activities from the life expectancy.
- The data for calculation is obtained from population surveys and period life table.
- The Sullivan's index collects mortality and disability data separately, and this data is almost often readily available.
- The Sullivan health expectancy reflects the current health of a real population adjusted for mortality levels and independent of age structure.

2

Determinants of Health

LONG ANSWER QUESTIONS

Q.1. a. List the effects of air pollution.
b. Explain the methods of control and prevention of air pollution. (7 + 8 = 15 Marks)

Q.2. a. Explain the steps in investigation of epidemic. (7 Marks)
b. Explain in detail the purification of water on a small scale. (8 Marks)

Q.3. a. Explain the effects of poor housing on health. (7 Marks)
b. Discuss the general measures that you will follow in controlling communicable diseases. (8 Marks)

Q.4. a. List out the sources of refuse.
b. Explain any four methods of disposal. (15 Marks)

Q.5. a. Explain the criteria of safe and wholesome water.
b. Describe the purification of water on large scale. (15 Marks)

SOLVED QUESTIONS PAPER

Q.1. a. List the effects of air pollution.
b. Explain the methods of control and prevention of air pollution.

(A) EFFECTS OF AIR POLLUTION

- **Respiratory and heart problems:** The effects of air pollution are alarming. Air pollution affects respiratory system causing breathing difficulties and diseases such as bronchitis, asthma, lung cancer, tuberculosis and pneumonia.
- **Global warming:** Another direct effect is the immediate alterations that the world is witnessing due to global warming. With increased temperatures worldwide, increase in sea levels and melting of ice from colder regions and icebergs, displacement and loss of habitat have already signaled an impending disaster if actions for preservation and normalization aren't undertaken soon.
- **Central nervous system:** Air pollution affects the central nervous system causing carbon monoxide (CO) poisoning. CO has more affinity for hemoglobin than oxygen and thus forms a stable compound carboxyhemoglobin (COHb), which is poisonous and causes suffocation and death.
- **Acid rain:** Harmful gases like nitrogen oxides and sulfur oxides are released into the atmosphere during the burning of fossil fuels. When it rains, the water droplets combines with these air pollutants, becomes acidic and then falls on the ground in the form of acid rain. Acid rain can cause great damage to human, animals and crops.
- **Eutrophication:** Eutrophication is a condition where high amount of nitrogen present in some pollutants gets developed on sea's surface and turns itself into algae and adversely affect fish, plants and animal species. The green colored algae that is present on lakes and ponds is due to presence of this chemical only.
- **Effect on wildlife:** Just like humans, animals also face some devastating effects of air pollution. Toxic chemicals present in the air can force wildlife species to move to new place and change their habitat. The toxic pollutants deposit over the surface of the water and can also affect sea animals.
- **Depletion of ozone layer:** Air pollution causes depletion of ozone layer due to which ultraviolet radiations can reach the earth and cause skin cancer, damage to eyes and immune system.
- **Other effects:** Air pollution from certain metals, pesticides and fungicides causes serious ailments.

- Lead pollution causes anemia, brain damage, convulsions and death.
- Certain metals cause problem in kidney, liver, circulatory system and nervous system.
- Fungicides cause nerve damage and death.
- Pesticides like DDT (Dichlorodiphenyltrichloroethane) which are toxic enter into our food chain and gets accumulated in the body causing kidney disorders and problems of brain and circulatory system.

(B) PREVENTION AND CONTROL OF AIR POLLUTION

Different techniques are used for controlling air pollution caused by 'gaseous pollutants' and that caused by 'particulate pollutants'.

- **Methods of controlling gaseous pollutants:** The air pollution caused by gaseous pollutants like hydrocarbons, sulfur dioxide, ammonia, carbon monoxide, etc. can be controlled by using three different methods: Combustion, Absorption and Adsorption.
    1. **Combustion:** This technique is applied when the pollutants are organic gases or vapors. The organic air pollutants are subjected to 'flame combustion or catalytic combustion' when they are converted to less harmful product carbon dioxide and a harmless product water.
    2. **Absorption:** In this method, the polluted air containing gaseous pollutants is passed through a scrubber containing a suitable liquid absorbent. The liquid absorbs the harmful gaseous pollutants present in air.
    3. **Adsorption:** In this method, the polluted air is passed through porous solid adsorbents kept in suitable containers. The gaseous pollutants are adsorbed at the surface of the porous solid and clean air passes through.
- **Methods of controlling particulate emissions:** The air pollution caused by particulate matter like dust, soot, ash, etc. can be controlled by using fabric filters, wet scrubbers, electrostatic precipitators and certain mechanical devices.
    - **Mechanical Devices:** It works on the basis of following:
        - **Gravity:** In this process, the particulate settle down by the action of gravitational force and get removed.
        - **Sudden change in the direction of air flow:** It brings about separation of particles due to greater momentum.

- **Fabric Filters:** The particulate matter is passed through a porous medium made of woven or filled fabrics.
  - The particulate present in the polluted air are filtered and gets collected in the fabric filters, while the gases are discharged.
  - The process of controlling air pollution by using fabric filters is called 'bag filtration'.
- **Wet Scrubbers:** They are used to trap SO_2, NH_3 and metal fumes by passing the fumes through water.
- **Electrostatic Precipitators:** When the polluted air containing particulate pollutants is passed through an electrostatic precipitator, it induces electric charge on the particles and then the aerosol particles get precipitated on the electrodes.

- Some other methods of controlling air pollution:
  - Tall chimneys should be installed in factories.
  - Better designed equipment and smokeless fuels should be used in homes and industries.
  - Renewable and non-polluting sources of energy like solar energy, wind energy, etc. should be used.
  - Automobiles should be properly maintained and adhere to emission control standards.
  - More trees should be planted along roadsides and houses.
- The **Air (Prevention and Control of Pollution) Act, 1981** is an Act of the Parliament of India to control and prevent air pollution. It was amended in 1987.

Q.2. a. Explain the steps in investigation of epidemic.
b. Explain in detail the purification of water on a small scale.

(A) STEPS IN INVESTIGATION OF EPIDEMIC

Once the decision to conduct a field investigation of an acute outbreak has been made, working quickly is essential—as is getting the right answer. In other words, epidemiologists cannot afford to conduct an investigation that is 'quick and dirty.' They must conduct investigations that are 'quick and clean.' Under such circumstances, epidemiologists find it useful to have a systematic approach to follow. This approach ensures that the investigation proceeds without missing important steps along the way.

Epidemiologic Steps of an Outbreak Investigation

1. **Prepare for field work:** Occasionally public health workers decide to conduct field investigation before confirming an increase in cases and verifying the diagnosis. More commonly, officials discover an increase in the number of cases of a particular disease and then decide that a field investigation is warranted. Preparation can be grouped into two categories:
   a. **Scientific and investigative issues**: Before departing, you should have a plan of action. What are the objectives of this investigation, i.e. what are you trying to accomplish? What will you do first, second, and third?
   b. **Management and operational issues**: A good field investigator must be a good manager and collaborator as well as a good epidemiologist, because most investigations are conducted by a team rather than just one individual. The team members must be selected before departure and know their expected roles and responsibilities in the field.
2. **Establish the existence of an outbreak**: An outbreak or an epidemic is the occurrence of more cases of disease than expected in a given area or among a specific group of people over a particular period of time. Usually, the cases are presumed to have a common cause or to be related to one another in some way.

   One of the first tasks of the field investigator is to verify that a cluster of cases is indeed an outbreak. Some clusters turn out to be true outbreaks with a common cause, some are sporadic and unrelated cases of the same disease and others are unrelated cases of similar but unrelated diseases.
3. **Verify the diagnosis**: The next step, verifying the diagnosis, is closely linked to verifying the existence of an outbreak. In fact, often these two steps are addressed at the same time. Verifying the diagnosis is important: (a) to ensure that the disease has been properly identified, since control measures are often disease-specific; and (b) to rule out laboratory error as the basis for the increase in reported cases.
4. **Construct a working case definition**: A case definition is a standard set of criteria for deciding whether an individual should be classified as having the health condition of interest. A case definition includes clinical criteria and—particularly in the setting of an outbreak investigation—restrictions by time,

place, and person. The clinical criteria should be based on simple and objective measures such as 'fever ≥ 40 °C (101 °F),' "three or more loose bowel movements per day, etc.

5. **Find cases systematically and record information**: Usually, the first effort to identify cases is directed at health care practitioners and facilities—physicians' clinics, hospitals, and laboratories—where a diagnosis is likely to be made. The data collection form should include the following types of information about each case.
   - **Identifying information:** For example, a name, address, and telephone number, etc.
   - **Demographic information:** For example age, sex, race, occupation.
   - **Clinical information:** Signs and symptoms allow investigators to verify that the case definition has been met.
   - **Risk factor information:** This information must be tailored to the specific disease in question.
   - **Reporter information.**
6. **Perform descriptive epidemiology**: Conceptually, the next step after identifying and gathering basic information on the persons with the disease is to systematically describe some of the key characteristics of those persons. This process, in which the outbreak is characterized by time, place, and person, is called descriptive epidemiology.

   This step is critical for several reasons.
   - Summarizing data by key demographic variables provides a comprehensive characterization of the outbreak—trends over time, geographic distribution (place), and the populations (persons) affected by the disease.
   - From this characterization, you can identify or infer the population at risk for the disease.
   - The characterization often provides clues about etiology, source, and modes of transmission that can be turned into testable hypotheses (see Step 7).
7. **Develop hypotheses:** Although the next conceptual step in an investigation is formulating hypotheses, in reality, investigators usually begin to generate hypotheses at the time of the initial telephone call. Depending on the outbreak, the hypotheses may address the source of the agent, the mode (and vehicle or vector) of transmission, and the exposures that caused the disease. The

hypotheses should be testable, since evaluating hypotheses is the next step in the investigation.

8. **Evaluate hypotheses epidemiologically**
9. **As necessary, reconsider, refine, and re-evaluate hypotheses:** When analytic epidemiology is unrevealing, rethink your hypotheses. Consider convening a meeting of the case-patients to look for common links or visiting their homes to look at the products on their shelves. Consider new vehicles or modes of transmission.
10. **Compare and reconcile with laboratory and/or environmental studies**: While epidemiology can implicate vehicles and guide appropriate public health action, laboratory evidence can confirm the findings. The laboratory was essential in both the outbreak of salmonellosis linked to marijuana and in the Legionellosis outbreak traced to the grocery store mist machine. The epidemiologic, environmental, and laboratory arms of the investigation complemented one another, and led to an inescapable conclusion, e.g. the well had been contaminated and was the source of the outbreak.
11. **Implement control and prevention measures**: Confidentiality is an important issue in implementing control measures. Health care workers need to be aware of the confidentiality issues relevant to collection, management and sharing of data. In general, control measures are usually directed against one or more segments in the chain of transmission (agent, source, mode of transmission, portal of entry, or host) that are susceptible to intervention, e.g. vaccinations promote development of specific antibodies that protect against infection, prophylactic use of antimalarial drugs, etc.
12. **Initiate and maintain surveillance**: Once control and prevention measures have been implemented, they must continue to be monitored. Reason is to monitor the situation and determine whether the prevention and control measures are working. Second, you need to know whether the outbreak has spread outside its original area or the area where the interventions were targeted. If so, effective disease control and prevention measures must be implemented in these new areas.
13. **Communicate findings:** Development of a communications plan and communicating with those who need to know during the investigation is critical. The final task is to summarize

the investigation, its findings, and its outcome in a report, and to communicate this report in an effective manner. This communication usually takes two forms: An oral briefing for local authorities and a written report.

(B) PURIFICATION OF WATER ON A SMALL SCALE

Household Methods of Purification

- **Boiling:** Boiling is the oldest and satisfactory method of purification of water on small scale. Boiling for 5 to 10 minutes kills bacteria, spores, cysts and ova of intestinal parasites. It also removes hardness of water and soft water is produced. Boiling is an excellent method of purification of water provided boiling is done in a neat and clean vessel and after boiling it is stored in clean covered container. Preferably water should be boiled in the same container in which it is to be stored. Only that much amount of water should be boiled which can be used within a few hours.
- **Chemicals:** Various types of chemical agents used for disinfection of water are discussed as follows:
  - **Bleaching powder (Chlorinated Lime):** Chemically it is $CaOCl_2$. Approximately 2.5 gm of a good quality of bleaching powder could be required to disinfect 1000 liters of water. Bleaching powder will not directly purify the turbid and polluted water. Therefore such water should first be treated with preliminary filtration and then subjected to chlorination.
  - **Chlorine tablets:** These tablets are good for disinfecting small quantities of water. They are available in different strengths for disinfecting various quantities of water. One tablet of 500 mg is sufficient for disinfecting 20 liters of water. These are available in the market under various trade names, e.g. halazone tablets manufactured by the Boots company.
  - **Alum:** Alum is not a germicidal. It is used to purify muddy water and to remove turbidity. 60 to 240 mg of alum can purify 4-5 liters of water. Calcium carbonate which is present in all kinds of water also gets precipitated as calcium sulfate and aluminum hydrate. The suspended impurities as well as bacteria also get precipitated which are removed after filtration and clear purified water is obtained.

  - **Potassium permanganate:** It is a strong oxidising agent and can kill cholera vibrios but it does not destroy other disease producing organisms. It is used for disinfecting wells. Its dose is 0.5 parts per million (0.5 ppm). It is not suitable for disinfecting large volume of water. Its disadvantages are that it alters the taste, smell and color of water thus treated. Moreover this method is not considered dependable therefore no longer used for disinfecting the water.
- **Domestic filters:** Water for drinking purposes can be purified by means of domestic filters which are discussed below:
  - **Berkefeld filters:** These are cylindrical filters known as 'filter candles' or 'ceramic candles'. They are made up of unglazed porcelain or kieselguhr and are available in various porosity grades. When water is purified through these candles, the pores get clogged, which need cleaning from time to time at least once a week by scrubbing with a hard brush and passing the water under pressure from inside to outside direction which will remove the entangled particles from the interstices.
  - **Pasteur-Chamberland filter:** It is made up of unglazed porcelain tubes which can be screwed on to a water tap. They work only under pressure and muddy water cannot be filtered through it because the pores will be immediately blocked.

    Therefore such water must be cleaned to remove mud. For cleaning the filters they are scrubbed from outside with a hard brush and water is made to pass under pressure from inside to outside. They are quick and reliable as they make the water free from all kinds of impurities including bacteria.

Disinfection of Wells

- **Simple chlorination:** There are steps involved in simple chlorination
  - **Calculating the amount of water in a well:** The formula for calculating the amount of water in a well is:
    Volume of water = [(3.14 × d × h)/4] × 1000 (liters)
    Here, d is the diameter of water, h is the depth of well.
  - **Determining the amount of bleaching powder:** Horrock's apparatus is used to calculate the amount of bleaching powder required for disinfection. For disinfection 1000

liters of water, 2.5 gm of good quality of bleaching powder is required.

- **Making solution of bleaching powder:** Bleaching powder is put into a bucket and made into a paste by adding little quantity of water. Then more water is added till the bucket is almost three fourth full of water. Solution is stirred and allowed to sediment at the bottom; due to this lime settles down. The water with chlorine is transferred to other bucket and the lime is thrown away.
- **Mixing of solution in water:** The bucket containing the chlorine solution is lowered into the well. After that well water is agitated by lowering and drawing up the bucket several times so that chlorine water is mixed properly with the well water. Contact period of 60 minutes should be allowed after chlorination.

- **Double pot method**: In this method two cylindrical pots are used. 1 kg bleaching powder and 2 kg sand is placed in the inner pot. This pot is placed in a circular outer pot. Both pots have a hole of 1 cm diameter. In case of inner pot, this hole is in the inner portion while in the case of outer pot, it is in the lower portion. Pots are closed at the upper portion and lowered into the well up to a depth of 1 meter and fixed at that level for some period. From the lower hole of the outer pot, chlorine continues to dissolve in water. Using this technique a well with a capacity of 4500 liters of water can be kept disinfected for a period of 2–3 weeks.

Q.3. a. Explain the effects of poor housing on health.
b. Discuss the general measures that you will follow in controlling communicable diseases.

(A) EFFECTS OF POOR HOUSING ON THE HEALTH

- **Overcrowding:** It is one of the many tangible impacts of housing crisis on households across the country. Overcrowded home have been linked with slow growth in children which correlated with an increased risk of heart disease as an adult. Research shows that children living in overcrowded homes are 10 times more likely to have meningitis and 3 times more likely to have respiratory problems.
- **Infectious disease**: Poor housing may include a contaminated water supply, poor waste disposal and insect and rodent

infestation, all of which have been shown to contribute to the spread of infectious disease. Tuberculosis and respiratory infections are the common diseases linked with overcrowded living.

- **Accidents:** Substandard housing has been associated with increased risk of injuries such as falls and burns. Common attributes of poor housing includes exposed heating sources, slippery surfaces, unprotected upper story windows, poorly designed stairs with inadequate lighting, etc.
- **Poor housing** leads to obstacle in the physical and mental development of an individual.
- **Chronic illness:** Indoor air quality and exposure to dampness are attributers to asthma and other allergic infections. It is hypothesized that damp environment are hospitable to mites, roaches, viruses and molds. Paints used in homes may be contaminated with lead, contributing to the neurodevelopment problems in the children.
- **Psychological effects**: Insufficient area and substandard of house may give rise to a feeling of inferiority and detachment.

(B) MEASURES FOR THE PREVENTION AND CONTROL OF COMMUNICABLE DISEASE

Controlling the Source or Reservoir of Infection

- **Surveillance:** Surveillance is defined as 'the continuous scrutiny (inspection) of the factors that determine the occurrence and distribution of disease and other conditions of ill-health'.
  The main objectives are:
  - To provide information about new and changing trends in the health status of a population, e.g. morbidity, mortality, nutritional status or other indicators and environmental hazards, health practices and other factors that may affect health.
  - To provide feedback which may be expected to modify the policy and the system itself and lead to redefinition of objectives.
  - Provide timely warning of public health disasters so that interventions can be mobilized.
- **Notification:** The purpose of notification is to take immediate measures against the spread of disease. As soon as the

information is received regarding communicable disease, it is the responsibility of the concerned person to notify the health and administrative officer. By timely notification, diseases can be checked, before it becomes an epidemic.
- **Isolation:** The purpose of isolation is to limit the spread of the disease in the community. The duration of isolation depends on the particular disease. Isolation can be standard, strict or protective.
- **Treatment:** Treatment reduces the communicability of disease by proper medication. Prompt treatment is an important aspect for the control of infectious disease.
- **Disinfection:** Proper destruction of the infectious agent in the excretions by the patient are important steps in preventing the spread of infection.

Blocking the Channels of Transmission

- Breaking the chain of infectious disease cycle
- Preventing the spread through 5 F`s
  - Food stuff
  - Fomites
  - Flies
  - Feces
  - Fingers

  For example, in malaria control, priority goes to the control of mosquitoes.

Protection of Susceptible Population

- **Immunization:** Before the onset of disease, susceptible people should be immunized. Booster doses are required to keep up the level of herd immunity.
- **Health education:** By educating general public and through their active participation we can successfully control the infectious disease. Emphasize the importance of proper food, housing, waste disposal and health habits.

Role of Community Health Nurse in Controlling the Spread of Infectious Disease

- Notification of infectious diseases to the concerned authority.
- Preventing sale of infected articles.
- Preventing infected people from using public transport.
- Cleaning and disinfection of premises.

- Administering immunization.
- Complete isolation of infected persons.
- Obtaining information from households and schools in order to prevent the spread of infectious diseases.
- Surveillance and analysis of trends in communicable disease.
- Liaison with key stakeholders involved in the control of infectious disease.
- Prevention, investigation, and control of health protection incidents including the prevention, investigation and control of outbreaks and incidents involving communicable diseases, chemical, radiological and other environmental hazards.
- Support the development and implementation of prevention and health promotion programs.
- Teaching and training of local health professionals in health protection.
- Creating mass awareness by educating community people regarding infectious disease, personal and environmental hygiene, importance of food hygiene, waste disposal, healthy habits, protection from arthropods borne disease, etc.

Q.4. a. List out the sources of refuse
b. Explain any four methods of disposal.

(A) SOURCES OF REFUSE

Sources of refuse are:

Source	*Typical waste generators*	*Types of wastes*
Residential	Single and multifamily dwellings	Food wastes, paper, cardboard, plastics, textiles, leather, yard wastes, wood, glass, metals, ashes, special wastes (e.g. bulky items, consumer electronics, white goods, batteries, oil, tires), and household hazardous wastes)
Industrial	Light and heavy manufacturing, fabrication, construction sites, power and chemical plants.	Housekeeping wastes, packaging, food wastes, construction and demolition materials, hazardous wastes, ashes, special wastes.
Commercial	Stores, hotels, restaurants, markets, office buildings, etc.	Paper, cardboard, plastics, wood, food wastes, glass, metals, special wastes, hazardous wastes.

Contd...

Contd...

Source	Typical waste generators	Types of wastes
Institutional	Schools, hospitals, prisons, government centers.	Same as commercial.
Construction and demolition	New construction sites, road repair, renovation sites, demolition of buildings.	Wood, steel, concrete, dirt, etc.
Municipal services	Street cleaning, landscaping, parks, beaches, other recreational areas, water and wastewater treatment plants.	Street sweepings; landscape and tree trimmings; general wastes from parks, beaches, and other recreational areas; sludge.
Process (manufacturing, etc.)	Heavy and light manufacturing, refineries, chemical plants, power plants, mineral extraction and processing.	Industrial process wastes, scrap materials, off-specification products, slay, tailings.
Agriculture	Crops, orchards, vineyards, dairies, feedlots, farms.	Spoiled food wastes, agricultural wastes, hazardous wastes (e.g. pesticides).

(B) METHODS OF DISPOSAL

Four methods of disposal are:

(i) Landfill

The landfill is the most popularly used method of waste disposal used today. This process of waste disposal focuses attention on burying the waste in the land. Landfills are found in all areas. There is a process used that eliminates the odors and dangers of waste before it is placed into the ground.

This method is becoming less these days although, thanks to the lack of space available and the strong presence of methane and other landfill gases, both of which can cause numerous contamination problems. Many areas are reconsidering the use of landfills.

(ii) Incineration/Combustion

Incineration or combustion is a type disposal method in which municipal solid wastes are burned at high temperatures so as to convert them into residue and gaseous products. The biggest advantage of this type of method is that it can reduce the volume of solid waste to 20 to 30 percent of the original volume, decreases the space they take up and reduce the stress on landfills. This process is also known as thermal treatment where solid waste materials are converted by incinerators into heat, gas, steam and ash.

(iii) Recovery and Recycling

Resource recovery is the process of taking useful discarded items for a specific next use. These discarded items are then processed to extract or recover materials and resources or convert them to energy in the form of useable heat, electricity or fuel.

Recycling is the process of converting waste products into new products to prevent energy usage and consumption of fresh raw materials. Recycling is the third component of Reduce, Reuse and Recycle waste hierarchy. The idea behind recycling is to reduce energy usage, reduce volume of landfills, reduce air and water pollution, reduce greenhouse gas emissions and preserve natural resources for future use.

(iv) Plasma Gasification

Plasma gasification is another form of waste management. Plasma is a primarily an electrically charged or a highly ionized gas. Lighting is one type of plasma which produces temperatures that exceed 12,600 °F. With this method of waste disposal, a vessel uses characteristic plasma torches operating at +10,000 °F which is creating a gasification zone till 3,000 °F for the conversion of solid or liquid wastes into a syngas.

Q.5. a. Explain the criteria of safe and wholesome water.
b. Describe the purification of water on large scale.

(A) CRITERIA OF SAFE AND WHOLESOME WATER

Safe and wholesome water is defined as that which is:

- Free from pathogenic agents
- Free from harmful chemical substances
- Pleasant to taste, colorless and odorless
- Usable for domestic purposes

If water does not fulfill the above criteria it is said to be polluted or contaminated. Water pollution is a growing hazard in many developing countries owing to human activity. It is not possible to provide positive health to the community without ample and safe drinking water.

(B) PURIFICATION OF WATER ON A LARGE SCALE

The aims of the treatment are to remove unwanted constituents in the water and to make it safe to drink or fit for a specific purpose in industry or medical applications. The component of a typical water purification system comprises one or all of the following measures:

Pretreatment:

- **Pumping and containment:** The majority of water must be pumped from its source or directed into pipes or holding tanks. To avoid adding contaminants to the water, this physical infrastructure must be made from appropriate materials and constructed so that accidental contamination does not occur.
- **Screening:** The first step in purifying surface water is to remove large debris such as sticks, leaves, rubbish and other large particles which may interfere with subsequent purification steps. Most deep groundwater does not need screening before other purification steps.
- **Storage:** Water from rivers may also be stored in bankside reservoirs for periods between a few days and many months to allow natural biological purification to take place. This is especially important if treatment is by slow sand filters. Storage reservoirs also provide a buffer against short periods of drought or to allow water supply to be maintained during transitory pollution incidents in the source river.
  - **Physical purification:** Most of the floating or suspended impurities settle down in 24 hours due to the influence of sunlight or gravity.
  - **Chemical purification:** Aerobic bacteria found in water oxidizes the organic substances in the presence of oxygen dissolved in water.
  - **Biological purification:** Number of pathogenic bacteria is reduced in the river water that is stored for 5–7 days.

Filtration

After separating most floc, the water is filtered as the final step to remove remaining suspended particles and unsettled floc. Filter is of two types, rapid sand filter and slow sand filter.

- **Rapid sand filters (Mechanical filter):** The most common type of filter is a rapid sand filter. Water moves vertically through sand which often has a layer of activated carbon oranthracite coal above the sand. The top layer removes organic compounds, which contribute to taste and odor. The space between sand particles is larger than the smallest suspended particles, so simple filtration is not enough. Most particles pass through surface layers but are trapped in pore spaces or adhere to sand particles. Effective filtration extends into the depth of the filter. This property of the filter is key to its operation: If the top layer of sand were to block all the particles, the filter would quickly clog.

To clean the filter, water is passed quickly upward through the filter, opposite the normal direction (called *backwashing*) to remove embedded particles. Prior to this step, compressed air may be blown up through the bottom of the filter to break up the compacted filter media to aid the backwashing process; this is known as *air scouring*. This contaminated water can be disposed of, along with the sludge from the sedimentation basin, or it can be recycled by mixing with the raw water entering the plant although this is often considered poor practice since it re-introduces an elevated concentration of bacteria into the raw water.

Some water treatment plants employ pressure filters. These work on the same principle as rapid gravity filters, differing in that the filter medium is enclosed in a steel vessel and the water is forced through it under pressure.

Types:
- **Gravity type:** Paterson`s filter
- **Pressure type:** Candy`s filter

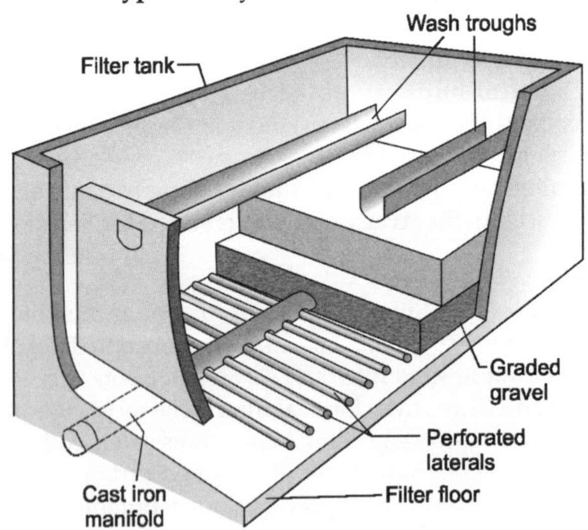

Advantages:

- Filters out much smaller particles than paper and sand filters can.
- Filters out virtually all particles larger than their specified pore sizes.
- They are quite thin and so liquids flow through them fairly rapidly.
- They are reasonably strong and so can withstand pressure differences across them of typically 2–5 atmospheres.
- They can be cleaned (back flushed) and reused.

• **Slow sand filters (Biological filters):** Slow sand filters may be used where there is sufficient land and space, as the water must be passed very slowly through the filters. These filters rely on biological treatment processes for their action rather than physical filtration. The filters are carefully constructed using graded layers of sand, with the coarsest sand, along with some gravel, at the bottom and finest sand at the top. Drains at the base convey treated water away for disinfection. Filtration depends on the development of a thin biological layer, called the zoogleal layer or schmutzdecke, on the surface of the filter.

An effective slow sand filter may remain in service for many weeks or even months if the pretreatment is well-designed and produces water with a very low available nutrient level which physical methods of treatment rarely achieve. Very low nutrient levels allow water to be safely sent through distribution systems with very low disinfectant levels, thereby reducing consumer irritation over offensive levels of chlorine and chlorine by-products. Slow sand filters are not backwashed; they are maintained by having the top layer of sand scraped off when flow is eventually obstructed by biological growth.

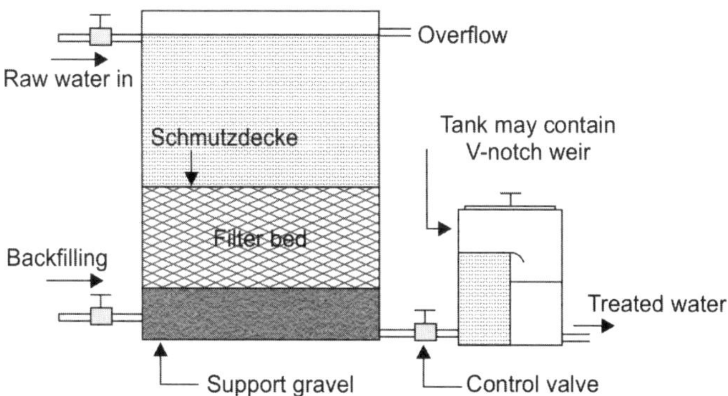

A specific 'large-scale' form of slow sand filter is the process of bank filtration, in which natural sediments in a riverbank are used to provide a first stage of contaminant filtration. While typically not clean enough to be used directly for drinking water, the water gained from the associated extraction wells is much less problematic than river water taken directly from the major streams where bank filtration is often used.

Removal of Ions and Other Dissolved Substances

- Ultrafiltration membranes use polymer membranes with chemically formed microscopic pores that can be used to filter out dissolved substances avoiding the use of coagulants. The type of membrane media determines how much pressure is needed to drive the water through and what sizes of micro-organisms can be filtered out.
- **Ion exchange:** Ion exchange systems use ion exchange resin- or zeolite-packed columns to replace unwanted ions. The most common case is water softening consisting of removal of Ca^{2+} and Mg^{2+} ions replacing them with benign (soap friendly) Na^{+} or K^{+} ions. Ion exchange resins are also used to remove toxic ions such as nitrite, lead, mercury, arsenic and many others.
- **Precipitative softening:** Water rich in hardness (calcium and magnesium ions) is treated with lime (calcium oxide) and/or soda-ash (sodium carbonate) to precipitate calcium carbonate out of solution utilizing the common on effect.
- **Electrodeionization:** Water is passed between a positive electrode and a negative electrode. Ion exchange membranes allow only positive ions to migrate from the treated water toward the negative electrode and only negative ions toward the positive electrode. High purity deionized water is produced continuously, similar to ion exchange treatment. Complete removal of ions from water is possible if the right conditions are met. The water is normally pre-treated with a reverse osmosis unit to remove non-ionic organic contaminants, and with gas transfer membranes to remove carbon dioxide.

Chlorination

It is the final step in the purification of water. It kills the harmful bacteria and makes it potable for drinking purposes. It acts as an oxidizing agent and oxidizes iron, manganese and hydrogen sulfide. Chlorine acts best as a germicide when pH value of water is around 7. Before chlorination chlorine demand of water should be estimated and it is defined as 'the amount of chlorine that is needed to destroy bacteria and to oxidize the organic matter present in the water'.

For disinfecting water, chlorine may be applied in one of the following forms:

- Chlorine gas
- Chloramine
- Perchloron or high test hypochlorite (HTH)
- Bleaching powder.

SHORT NOTES

(5 Marks)

Q.1. Food hygiene

Q.2. Pasteurization

Q.3. Food adulteration

Q.4. Primary health center

Q.5. Good housing

Q.6. Town planning

Q.7. Disposal of solid waste

Q.8. Oxidation pond

Q.9. Food fortification

Q.10. Meat hygiene

Q.11. PFA

1. FOOD HYGIENE

Food hygiene implies hygiene in the production, handling, distribution and serving of all type of food. Food safety is a scientific discipline describing handling, preparation, and storage of food in ways that prevent food borne illness. This includes a number of routines that should be followed to avoid potentially severe health hazards.

Food can transmit disease from person to person as well as serve as a growth medium for bacteria that can cause food poisoning. In developed countries there are intricate standards for food preparation, whereas in lesser developed countries the main issue is simply the availability of adequate safe water, which is usually a critical item. In theory, food poisoning is 100% preventable.

The five key principles of food hygiene, according to WHO, are:

1. Prevent contaminating food with pathogens spreading from people, pets, and pests.
2. Separate raw and cooked foods to prevent contaminating the cooked foods.
3. Cook foods for the appropriate length of time and at the appropriate temperature to kill pathogens.
4. Store food at the proper temperature.
5. Do use safe water and raw materials.

Points to be Kept in Mind Regarding Food Hygiene

- Sterilization of milk by boiling is a good method for domestic use. Choose processed foods for safety such as pasteurized milk.
- Wash your hands before handling food and often during food preparation.
- Hand washing is one of the most effective defenses against the spread of food borne illnesses.
- Separate raw meat, poultry and seafood from other foods as they contain microbes which can be transferred onto other foods during storage and food preservation.
- Don't keep cooked food at room temperature for more than 2 hours.
- Cook thoroughly especially meat, poultry, eggs and seafood.
- Don't consume food beyond their expiry date.
- Raw vegetables should be properly washed before cutting.

2. PASTEURIZATION

Definition: 'The heating of milk to such temperatures and for such periods of time as are required to destroy any pathogens that may be present while causing minimal changes in the composition, flavor and nutritive value.'

—An Expert Committee of WHO.

It was invented by French scientist **Louis Pasteur** during the nineteenth century. In 1864, Pasteur discovered that heating beer and wine was enough to kill most of the bacteria that caused spoilage, preventing these beverages from turning sour. The process achieves this by eliminating pathogenic microbes and lowering microbial numbers to prolong the quality of the beverage.

Methods of Pasteurization

- **Holder (Vat):** In this method, milk is heated and kept at 63–66 °C for 30 minutes and then quickly cooled to below 5 °C.
- **High temperature short time (HTST):** Milk is forced between metal plates or through pipes heated on the outside by hot water, and the milk is heated to 72 °C (161 °F) for 15 seconds. Milk simply labeled 'pasteurized' is usually treated with the HTST method.
- **Ultra high treating (UHT)**: In this method processing holds the milk at a temperature of 140 °C (284 °F) for four seconds. During UHT processing milk is sterilized and not pasteurized. The process is achieved by spraying the milk or juice through a nozzle into a chamber filled with high-temperature steam under pressure. After the temperature reaches 140 °C the fluid is cooled instantly in a vacuum chamber, and packed in a pre-sterilized airtight container.
- **Extended shelf life (ESL)**: Milk has a microbial filtration step and lower temperatures than UHT milk. Since 2007, it is no longer a legal requirement in European countries (for example in Germany) to declare ESL milk as ultra-heated; consequently, it is now often labeled as 'fresh milk' and just advertised as having an 'extended shelf life,' making it increasingly difficult to distinguish ESL milk from traditionally pasteurized fresh milk.

Test on Milk

- **Methylene blue reduction test:** For accepting milk to be accepted for pasteurization.
- **Phosphatase test:** To know efficacy of pasteurization.
- **Coli form test:** To know efficacy of pasteurization.
- **Standard plate test:** To know efficacy of pasteurization.

The Effect of Pasteurization on Nutrients and Flavor

Pasteurization can affect the nutrient composition and flavor of foods. In the case of milk, for example, the high-temperature, short-time treatments (HTST) cause less damage to the nutrient composition and sensory characteristics of foods than do the low-temperature, long-time treatments (LTLT).

Foods that are Commonly Pasteurized

- **Whole eggs removed from shells and sold as a liquid:** Large quantities of eggs are sold to restaurants and institutions out of the shell. The yolk and whole-egg products are pasteurized in their raw form. The egg white is pasteurized in its raw form if it is sold as a liquid or frozen product.

- **Dried eggs**: If eggs are sold dried, the egg white with the glucose removed is normally heat-treated in the container by holding it for 7 days in a hot room at a minimum temperature of 130 °F (54 °C).
- **Whole eggs pasteurized in the shell:** Egg whites coagulate at 140 °F (60 °C). Therefore, heating an egg above 140 °F would cook the egg, so processors pasteurize the egg in the shell at a low temperature, 130°F (54 °C), for a long time, 45 minutes. This new process is being used by some manufacturers, but it is not yet widely available. Pasteurizing eggs reduces the risk of contamination from pathogenic bacteria, such as *Salmonella,* which can cause severe illness and even death.
- **Milk:** Pasteurization improves the quality of milk and milk products and gives them a longer shelf life by destroying undesirable enzymes and spoilage bacteria. For example, the liquid is heated to 145 °F (63 °C) for at least 30 minutes or at least 161 °F (72 °C) for 15 seconds.
- **Today,** many foods, such as eggs, milk, juices, spices and ice cream, are pasteurized. Temperatures and times vary, depending on the product and the target organism.

3. FOOD ADULTERATION

It is defined as the process by which the quality or the nature of a given substance is reduced through the addition of a foreign or an inferior substance and the removal of a vital element.

Types of Adulterants

- **Intentional adulterants**: These are those substances that are added as a deliberate act on the part of the adulterer with the intention to increase the margin of profit, e.g. sand, marble chips, stones, mud, chalk powder, water, dyes, etc. These adulterants cause harmful effects on the body.
- **Incidental adulterants**: These adulterants are found in food substances due to ignorance, negligence or lack of proper facilities. It is not a willful act on the part of the adulterer, e.g. pesticides, droppings of rodents, larvae in food.
- **Metallic contamination**: Metallic contamination: Arsenic from pesticides, lead from water, mercury from effluent of chemical industries, tins from cans.

- **Packaging Hazards**: Polyethylene, polyvinyl chloride and allied compounds are used to produce flexible packaging material.

An Article of Food shall be Deemed to be Adulterated

- If the article sold by a vendor is not of the nature, substance or quality demanded by the purchaser and is to his prejudice, or is not of the nature, substance or quality which it purports or is represented to be
- If the article contains any other substance which affects, or if the article is so processed as to affect, injuriously the nature, substance or quality thereof
- If any inferior or cheaper substance has been substituted wholly or in part for the article so as to affect injuriously the nature, substance or quality thereof
- If any constituent of the article has been wholly or in part abstracted so as to affect injuriously the nature, substance or quality thereof
- If the article had been prepared, packed or kept under insanitary conditions whereby it has become contaminated or injurious to health
- If the article consists wholly or in part of any filthy, putrefied, rotten, decomposed or diseased animal or vegetable substance or is insect-infested or is otherwise unfit for human consumption
- If the article is obtained from a diseased animal
- If the article contains any poisonous or other ingredient which renders it injurious to health
- If the container of the article is composed, whether wholly or in part, of any poisonous or deleterious substance which renders its contents injurious to health
- If any coloring matter other than that prescribed in respect thereof is present in the article, or if the amounts of the prescribed coloring matter which is present in the article are not within the prescribed limits of variability
- If the article contains any prohibited preservative or permitted preservative in excess of the prescribed limits
- If the quality or purity of the article falls below the prescribed standard or its constituents are present in quantities not within the prescribed limits of variability, but which renders it injurious to health;
- If the quality or purity of the article falls below the prescribed standard or its constituents are present in quantities not within the prescribed limits of variability but which does not render it injurious to health:

Food Items with Type of Adulteration

S.No.	Item	Adulteration
1	Baking powder	Citric Acid
2	Non-alcoholic beverages	Non-permitted colors, saccharin, dulcin, lead, arsenic copper
3	Spices	Coal tar dyes, sand, grit, saw dust, lead chromate in turmeric, stalky and woody matter in zeera
4	Saffron	Colored dried tendril of maize cob
5	Honey	Water, sugar
6	Starchy foods	Sand, grit, foreign starches in arrowroot, etc.
7	Sugar	Chalk powder
8	Ice cream	Washing powder
9	Coffee and Tea	Husk, coal tar dyes, exhausted stuff, sand, grit, used tea dust
10	Milk	Urea, water, starch, fat removal
11	Ground nuts	Aflatoxin
12	Vanaspati	Animal fat, excessive hydrogenation, foreign flavor
13	Mustard seed	Argemone seeds
14	Oils	Argemone oil, mineral and castor oil
15	Pulses	Khesari dal, clay, stone, gravel
16	Salt	White powder, stone, rava

S.No.	Adulterant	Food commonly involved	Diseases or health effects
	Adulterants in food		
1.	Argemone seeds Argemone oil	Mustard seeds Edible oils and fats	Epidemic dropsy, Glaucoma, Cardiac arrest
2.	Artificially colored foreign seeds	As a substitute for cumin seed, poppy seed, black pepper	Injurious to health
	Chemical contamination		
3.	Mineral oil (white oil, petroleum fractions)	Edible oils and fats, Black pepper	Cancer
4.	Lead chromate	Turmeric whole and powdered, mixed spices	Anemia, abortion, paralysis, brain damage
	Bacterial contamination		
5.	Bacillus cereus	Cereal products, custards, puddings, sauces	Food infection (nausea, vomitting, abdominal pain, diarrhea)
6.	Salmonella spp.	Meat and meat products, raw vegetables, salads, shell-fish, eggs	Salmonellosis (food infection usually with fever and chills)

Some Adulterated Food Products and Their Adverse Effects

- **Turmeric, dals and pulses such as moong or channa:** Here adulterant is Metanil Yellow and Khesari Dal (Added to enhance the yellow color of a food substance). Its harmful effect is that it is highly carcinogenic and if consumed over a continuous period of time it can also cause stomach disorders.
- **Green chilies, green peas and other vegetables:** Here adulterant is Malachite Green (To accentuate the bright, glowing green color of the vegetable). Argemone seeds (used to add bulk and weight) that it is a colored dye that has proven to be carcinogenic for humans if consumed over a long period of time.
- **Mustard seeds and mustard oil:** Here adulterant is Argemone seeds (used to add bulk and weight). Papaya seeds (used to add bulk) that the consumption of these could cause epidemic dropsy and severe glaucoma. Young children and senior citizens with poor immunity are more susceptible to this.
- **Paneer, khoya, condensed milk and milk:** Here adulterant is starch (used to give it thick, rich texture). Its harmful effect is that it is unhygienic, unprocessed water and starch can cause stomach disorders. Starch greatly reduces the nutritional value of the ingredient.
- **Ice cream:** Here adulterant is pepperonil, ethyl acetate, butyraldehyde, ethyl acetate, nitrate, washing powder, etc. which are not less than poison. Pepper oil is used as a pesticide and ethylacetate causes terrible diseases affecting lungs, kidneys and heart.
- **Black pepper:** Here adulterant is Papaya seeds (used to add bulk). Its harmful effect is that Papaya seeds can cause serious liver problems and stomach disorders.

Law against Food Adulteration

- **FSSAI:** It establishes a new national regulatory body, the Food Safety and Standards Authority of India (hereinafter referred to as 'FSSAI'), to develop science based standards for food and to regulate and monitor the manufacture, processing, storage, distribution, sale and import of food so as to ensure the availability of safe and wholesome food for human consumption.

  Key Regulations of FSSA:
  - Packaging and labeling

- Signage and customer notices
- Licensing, registration and health and sanitary permits

- **Prevention of Food Adulteration Act**: The Prevention of Food Adulteration Bill was passed by both the house of Parliament and received the assent of the President on 29th September, 1954. It came into force on 1st June, 1955 as The Prevention of Food Adulteration Act, 1954 (37 of 1954). See details in Q.No 11.

4. PRIMARY HEALTH CENTER

Primary health center are state-owned rural health care facilities in India. They are essentially single-physician clinics usually with facilities for minor surgeries, too. They are part of the government-funded public health system in India and are the most basic units of this system. Primary health care is the first level of contact of the individual, the family and the community with the national health services.

Definition: 'Primary health care is essential health care made universally accessible to individuals and acceptable to them, through their full participation and at a cost that the community and country can afford' —*The Alma Ata Conference*

Elements of Primary Health Care

According to Alma Ata Declaration, Primary health care includes at least 8 elements; they are:

1. Education of the people about prevailing health problems and methods of preventing and controlling them.
2. Promotion of food supply and proper nutrition.
3. Adequate supply of safe water and basic sanitation.
4. Maternal and child health care and family planning.
5. Immunization against major infectious diseases.
6. Prevention and control of locally endemic diseases.
7. Appropriate treatment of common diseases and injuries.
8. Provision of essential drugs.

Principles of Primary Health Care

WHO (1984) Expert Committee recognized that there are five principles of Primary Health Care.

1. **Equitable distribution:** Equitable distribution of health services to all sections of society.
2. **Community involvement:** Community must participate in the planning, implementation and maintenance of health services.

3. **Appropriate technology:** Low cost treatment should be used by the clinician.
4. **Focus on prevention:** Main focus should be on the prevention aspect.
5. **Multisectoral approach:** Along with the health sector, other sectors should be involved such as education, agriculture, etc.

Focus

- Regular medical checkup
- **Infant immunization programs:** Immunization for newborns under the national immunization program is dispensed through the PHCs. This program is fully subsidized.
- **Anti-epidemic programs:** The PHCs act as the primary epidemic diagnostic and control centers for the rural India. Whenever a local epidemic breaks out, the system's doctors are trained for diagnosis. They identify suspected cases and refer for further treatment.
- **Birth control programs:** Services under the national birth control programs are dispensed through the PHCs. Sterilization surgeries such as vasectomy and tubectomy are done here. These services, too, are fully subsidized.
- **Pregnancy and related care:** A major focus of the PHC system is medical care for pregnancy and child birth in rural India. This is because people from rural India resist approaching doctors for pregnancy care which increases neonatal death. Hence, pregnancy care is a major focus area for the PHCs.
- **Emergencies:** All the PHCs store drugs for medical emergencies which could be expected in rural areas. For example, antivenoms for snake bites, rabies vaccinations, etc.

Functions

The Government of India's initiative to create and expand the presences of Primary Health Centers throughout the country is consistent with the eight elements of primary health care outlined in the Alma Ata declaration. These are listed below:

1. Provision of medical care
2. Maternal-child health including family planning
3. Safe water supply and basic sanitation
4. Prevention and control of locally endemic diseases
5. Collection and reporting of vital statistics
6. Education about health

7. National health programs, as relevant referral services
8. Training of health guides, health workers, local dais and health assistants basic laboratory workers

5. GOOD HOUSING

Good-quality housing is a key element for ensuring a healthy village. Poor housing can lead to many health problems, and is associated with infectious diseases (such as tuberculosis), stress and depression. Everyone should therefore have access to good-quality housing and a pleasant home environment that makes them happy and content.

Characteristics and features of ideal house:

- An idyllic house should meet the physical and social needs of the family. It must be equipped with:
  - A kitchen to cook food and a dining room to eat and enjoy meals or even snacks.
  - Bedroom where the each member can able to rest, sleep and unwind, and have a sense of privacy.
  - A bathroom to meet the personal necessities of the family.
  - A living room to host guests.
  - A garden and lawn where they can plant and grow trees, vegetables, and ornamental plants, and can be a good place where kids can play and have some fun.
  - The rooms in the house should be planned well as all areas utilized in connected activities near to each other.
  - The kitchen should be near the dining room to allow foods being served easily during mealtime.
  - The living room should be near the dining room to allow the guests to be served easily during meal time.
  - The bathroom should be adjoined to the bedrooms for personal necessities.
  - The washing area should be positioned at the back of the house so that the clothes will be hanged in the clothes lines with relative ease.
- Rooms in the house should neither be too small nor too big, but spacious enough.
- There should be wide enough windows for proper ventilation and lighting will aid in contributing to the family's good health.
- It should have sufficient supply of water for mundane tasks such as laundering, bathing and other personal needs of the family.

- Work areas should be planned to prevent crowded space and walking back and forth from one place to another.

6. TOWN PLANNING

Town planning is a technical and political process concerned with the use of land, protection and use of the environment, public welfare, and the design of the urban environment, including air, water, and the infrastructure passing into and out of urban areas such as transportation, communications, and distribution networks. Urban planning is also referred to as **urban and regional**, **regional**, **town**, **city**, **rural planning** or some combination in various areas worldwide. Urban planning takes many forms and it can share perspectives and practices with urban design.

Objectives of Town Planning

- Providing basic amenities to the citizens such as safe water supply, healthful housing, appropriate lightening, medical facilities, etc.
- Proving good transport system.
- Conservation of environment by controlling air, water, noise, soil pollution.
- Having proper disposal of waste management.
- Proving welfare services to the public, e.g. Parks, swimming pool, amusement centers, etc.

Urban planning guides and ensures the orderly development of settlements and satellite communities which commute into and out of urban areas or share resources with it. Urban planners in the field are concerned with research and analysis, strategic thinking, architecture, urban design, public consultation, policy recommendations, implementation and management.

Basic Principles of Town Planning

The basic principles of city planning considered from the technical, economical and the administration point of view are as follows:

- The scope of city planning consists of principally in fixing the baselines of all traffic movements and transit facilities, including streets, railroads and canals. These transit facilities have to be treated liberally and systematically.
- The street network should be planned in such a way that the main streets with the existing streets have to be given greater

consideration. The auxiliary streets have to be fixed based on local conditions, and in addition, other subordinate streets have to be treated in accordance with the necessities of the immediate future, or with a wish of placing their development in the hands of interested property owners.

- Some parts of the city have to be grouped in accordance with the location of the part and individual characteristics. These parts may be subjected to such modifications as may be demanded by the sanitary considerations and the exigencies of commerce and industry.
- The building departments have to adhere to by some rights and privileges related to fire protection; freedom from interference; health and safety of buildings and all aesthetic considerations.
- The town or city municipal authorities have to facilitate for legal measures in cases of expropriation and impropriation and should also create a law providing for the regulation of the contour of new or reconstructed blocks to be built upon.
- The property holders, who are directly benefited by improvements, have to reimburse the city by paying funds in advance to the city for such a purpose. It is advisable to fix the normal cost per front foot and collect the amount stipulated before the work is begun.
- The municipality has to constantly supervise the activities of interested property owners associations, in regard to the improvement of certain sections.
- Efficient use of land and infrastructure: Land upon which it is necessary to make improvements should only be built upon under reservations for its subsequent use by the city. High-density development, infill development, redevelopment and the adaptive re-use of existing buildings result in efficient utilization of land resources and more compact urban areas.

7. DISPOSAL OF SOLID WASTE

Answer: Rapid population growth and urbanization in developing countries has led to people generating enormous quantities of solid waste and consequent environmental degradation. The waste is normally disposed in open dumps creating nuisance and environmental degradation. Solid wastes cause a major risk to public health and the environment. Management of solid wastes is important in order to minimize the adverse effects posed by their indiscriminate disposal.

Types of Solid Wastes

Depending on the nature of origin, solid wastes are classified into:

- **Urban or municipal wastes:** Urban waste classified into biodegradable (e.g. food, vegetable, tea leaves, etc.) and non-biodegradable waste (e.g. polythene bags, glass bottles, etc).
- **Industrial wastes:** The main sources of industrial wastes are chemical industries, metal and mineral processing industries.
- **Hazardous wastes:** Solid waste management involves waste generation, mode of collection, transportation, segregation of wastes and disposal techniques.

Methods of Solid Wastes Disposal

- **Burning:** Refused is collected in an open space and burned every day.
- **Encapsulation:** Cement-lined pits or high-density plastic containers or drums are filled to 75% capacity with health care waste. The container is then filled with plastic foam, sand, cement, or clay to immobilize the waste. The encapsulated waste is then disposed of in a landfill or left in place if the container is constructed in the ground.
- **Sanitary landfill or controlled tipping:** Solid wastes are placed in a sanitary landfill in which alternate layers of 80 cm thick refuse is covered with selected earth-fill of 20 cm thickness. After 2–3 years, solid waste volume shrinks by 25–30% and land is used for parks, roads and small buildings. This is the most common and cheapest method of waste disposal and is mostly employed in Indian cities. The main disadvantage is that it requires proper planning, design and operation.
- **Plasma gasification:** Plasma gasification is another form of waste management. Plasma is a primarily an electrically charged or a highly ionized gas. Lighting is one type of plasma which produces temperatures that exceed 12,600 °F . With this method of waste disposal, a vessel uses characteristic plasma torches operating at +10,000 °F which is creating a gasification zone till 3,000 °F for the conversion of solid or liquid wastes into a syngas. This form of waste disposal provides renewable energy and an assortment of other fantastic benefits.
- **Incineration:** An incinerator is a unit or facility used to burn trash and other types of waste until it is reduced to ash. An incinerator is constructed of heavy, well-insulated materials, so that it does not give off extreme amounts of external heat.

The high levels of heat are kept inside the furnace or unit so that the waste is burned quickly and efficiently. If the heat were allowed to escape, the waste would not burn as completely or as rapidly. Incineration is a disposal method in which solid organic wastes are subjected to combustion so as to convert them into residue and gaseous products. This method is useful for disposal of residue of both solid waste management and solid residue from waste water management. This process reduces the volumes of solid waste to 20 to 30% of the original volume.

- **Composting**: It is another popular method practiced in many cities in our country. In this method, bulk organic waste is converted into fertilizer by biological action. Separated compostable waste is dumped in underground trenches in layers of 1.5 m and finally covered with earth of 20 cm and left for decomposition. Sometimes, actinomycetes are introduced for active decomposition. Within 2 to 3 days biological action starts. Organic matter is destroyed by actinomycetes and lot of heat is liberated increasing the temperature of compost by 75 °C and the refuse is finally converted into powdery brown colored odorless mass called humus that has a fertilizing value and can be used in agriculture. Humus contains lot of Nitrogen essential for plant growth apart from phosphates and other minerals.

  There are two methods of composting:

  1. **Anaerobic method (Bangalore method):** It is an anaerobic method. The earthen trenches 10 × 1.5 × 1.5 m – left for decomposition – takes 4 to 5 months
  2. **Aerobic method (Mechanical method):** Process of stabilization is expedited by mechanical devices of turning the compost. Compost is stabilized in about 1 to 2 weeks. To enrich compost – night soil, cow dung, etc. are added to the refuse. Usually done in compost pits. Arrangements for draining of excess moisture are provided at the base of the pit. At the bottom of the pit, a layer of ash, ground limestone, or loamy soil is placed – to neutralize acidity in the compost material and providing an alkaline medium for microorganisms. The pit is filled by alternate layers of refuse (laid in layers of depth 30–40 cm) and night soil or cow dung (laid over it in a thin layer). Material is turned every 5 days or so. After approximately 30 days – it is ready for use.

- Composting is one of the best method of waste disposal as it can turn unsafe organic products into safe compost. Manure added to soil increases water retention and ion-exchange capacity of soil. This method can be used to treat several industrial solid wastes. Manure can be sold thereby reducing cost of disposing wastes. On the other side, it is slow process and takes lot of space.

8. OXIDATION POND

Oxidation pond uses a natural process for wastewater treatment that employs a combination of macrophytic plants, substrates and microorganisms in a more or less artificial pond to treat wastewater. It is also known as stabilization ponds, lagoons or waste management ponds. The technique is frequently used to treat municipal wastewater, industrial effluent, municipal run-off or stormwater. After treatment, the effluent may be returned to surface water or reused as irrigation water (or reclaimed water) if the effluent quality is high enough.

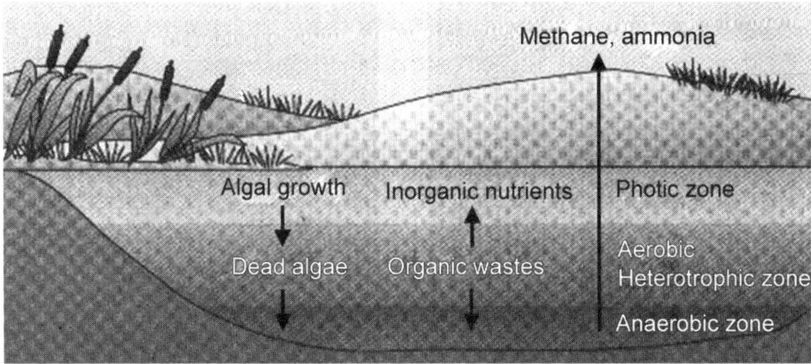

Stabilization ponds are commonly used for wastewater treatment in developing countries. Types of treatment ponds include anaerobic lagoons, facultative pond and aerated lagoons.

- **Anaerobic lagoons:** It is the first pond in the treatment system. By definition, anaerobic pond is devoid of oxygen. This encourages the growth of anaerobic bacteria which breakdown the solid content of the effluent. Anaerobic lagoons are created from a manure slurry, which is washed out from underneath the animal pens and then piped into the lagoon. Sometimes the slurry is placed in an intermediary holding tank under or next to the barns before it is deposited in a lagoon. Once in the lagoon, the manure settles into two layers: Solid, or sludge, layer and the liquid layer. The manure then undergoes the process of anaerobic respiration, whereby the volatile organic compounds are converted into carbon dioxide and methane. Anaerobic lagoons are usually used to pretreat high strength industrial wastewaters, and municipal wastewaters. This allows for preliminary sedimentation of suspended solids as a pretreatment process.

- **Aerobic pond(s):** An **aerated lagoon** or **aerated basin** is a holding and/or treatment pond provided with artificial aeration to promote the biological oxidation of wastewaters. There are many other biological processes for treatment of wastewaters, for example, activated sludge, trickling filters, rotating biological contactors and biofilters. They all have in common the use of oxygen (or air) and microbial action to biotreat the pollutants in wastewaters.
- **Facultative lagoons** are a type of stabilization pond used for biological treatment of industrial and domestic wastewater. Sewage or organic waste from food or fiber processing may be catabolized in a system of constructed ponds where adequate space is available to provide an average waste retention time exceeding a month. A series of ponds prevents mixing of untreated waste with treated wastewater and allows better control of waste residence time for uniform treatment efficiency.

9. FOOD FORTIFICATION

Food fortification refers to the addition of micronutrients to processed foods.

In many situations, this strategy can lead to relatively rapid improvements in the micronutrient status of a population, and at a very reasonable cost. Fortification of food with micronutrients is a valid technology for reducing micronutrient malnutrition as part of a food-based approach when and where existing food supplies and limited access fail to provide adequate levels of the respective nutrients in the diet. Food fortification was identified as the second strategy of four by the WHO and FAO to begin decreasing the incidence of nutrient deficiencies at the global level.

Ideally, a fortified food should:

- Be commonly consumed by the target population
- Have a constant consumption pattern with a low-risk of excess consumption

- Have good stability during storage
- Be relatively low in cost
- Be centrally processed with minimal stratification of the fortificant
- Have no interaction between the fortificant and the carrier food
- Be contained in most meals with availability unrelated to socio-economic status
- Be linked to energy intake.

Selection of an appropriate vehicle is a critical step in successful fortification.

General Principles for Addition of Nutrients to Foods

Within the FAO/WHO food standards program, the Codex Alimentarius Commission has adopted 'General Principles for the Addition of Essential Nutrients to Foods'. The basic principles for the addition of essential nutrients to foods, as stated by the Codex Alimentarius Commission are:

- The essential nutrient should be present at a level which will not result in either an excessive or an insignificant intake of the added essential nutrient considering amounts from other sources in the diet.
- The addition of an essential nutrient to a food should not result in an adverse effect on the metabolism of any other nutrient.
- The essential nutrient should be sufficiently stable in the food under customary conditions of packaging, storage, distribution and use.
- The essential nutrient should be biologically available from the food.
- The essential nutrient should not impart undesirable characteristics to the food and should not unduly shorten the food shelf life.
- Technology and processing facilities should be available to permit the addition of the essential nutrient in a satisfactory manner.
- Addition of essential nutrients to foods should not be used to mislead or deceive the consumer as to the nutritional merit of the food.
- The additional cost should be reasonable for the intended consumer.
- Methods of measuring, controlling and/or enforcing the levels of added essential nutrients in the foods should be available.

- When provision is made in food standards, regulations or guidelines, for the addition of essential nutrients to foods, specific provisions should be included identifying the essential nutrients which are to be considered or be required and the levels at which they should be present in the food to achieve their intended purposes.

Types of Fortification

- **Mass fortification** is when micronutrients are added to foods commonly consumed by the mass population – such as cereals and condiments.
- **Universal fortification** is when micronutrients are added to food consumed by animals as well as people, such as with iodization of salt.
- **Targeted fortification** exists in such areas as school food programs, when, for example, a cracker is specifically fortified for a targeted age group.

Examples of Fortification in Foods

- **Iodized salt:** Salt is high in sodium and is used on many different foods to add flavor. It is also fortified with iodine. 'Iodized' salt benefits thyroid function.
- **Folic acid:** Folic acid functions in reducing blood homocysteine levels, forming red blood cells, proper growth and division of cells, and preventing neural tube defects (NTDs).
- **Sterols and stanols:** Sterols and stanols are naturally-occurring substances found in various plant and animal cells. Sterols and stanols can help those with high cholesterol. According to the Cleveland Clinic, consuming 1.3 to 3.4 grams of sterols and stanols a day can significantly reduce cholesterol. Foods that are fortified with substances include yogurt, margarine, chocolate, cheese, granola bars and orange juice.
- **Bread:** Bread is composed of whole grains or white flour and it is often fortified with folic acid, a B-vitamin also known as 'folate.'
- **Soy milk:** Soy milk is derived from soy beans and it is used as an alternative to regular milk by people who have allergies or are strict vegetarians. It is high in protein and is often fortified with calcium, which it does not naturally contain.
- **Refined grains have B-vitamins and iron:** Most grains and grain products have been fortified with thiamin, or vitamin

B-1; riboflavin, or vitamin B-2; niacin, or vitamin B-3; and iron. These products include bread, corn meal, flour, pasta and rice.

- **Fortified milk provides vitamin D:** Milk is not a natural source of vitamin D, but fortified milk is a main source of vitamin D. Other foods often fortified with vitamin D include milk substitutes, such as fortified soy milk, fortified orange juice and fortified breakfast cereals. Fortified milk also provides vitamin A.

10. MEAT HYGIENE

Meat processing hygiene is part of Quality Management (QM) of meat plants and refers to the hygienic measures to be taken during the various processing steps in the manufacture of meat products. Regulatory authorities usually provide the compulsory national framework for food/meat hygiene programs through laws and regulations and monitor the implementation of such laws. At the meat industry level, it is the primary responsibility of individual enterprises to develop and apply efficient meat hygiene programs specifically adapted to their relevant range of production.

The meat borne diseases are:

- **Tapeworm:** *Taenia solium, Taenia saginata, Trichinella spiralis,* etc.
- **Bacterial:** Anthrax, Actinomycosis, Tuberculosis, Food poisoning.

Signs of a Good Meat

- **Color:** Color should not be pale pink or deep purple.
- **Touch:** Meat should be firm and elastic to touch. It should not be greasy or slimy.
- **Odor:** The odor should be agreeable.

Principles of Meat Hygiene

There are three principles of meat hygiene, which are crucial for meat processing operations.

- **Prevent microbial contamination** of raw materials, intermediate (semi-manufactured) goods and final products during meat product manufacture through absolute cleanliness of tools, working tables, machines as well as hands and outfits of personnel.
- **Minimize microbial growth** in raw materials, semi-manufactured goods and final products by storing them at a low temperature.

- **Reduce** or **eliminate microbial contamination** by applying heat treatment at the final processing stage for extension of shelf life of products (except dried and fermented final products, which are shelf-stable through low A_w and pH)

For the sanitary quality and safety related to meat processing, two useful schemes can be applied known as

1. **Good Hygienic Practices (GHP)** and
2. **Hazard Analysis and Critical Control Point (HACCP) Scheme**.

Good Hygienic Practices (GHP): It follows general hygienic rules and applies recognized hygienic principles as well as laws and regulations issued by the competent authorities, referring to meat and meat products, equipment, premises and personnel. GHP schemes are **not factory specific,** they apply to all types of meat plants. They are intended to establish and maintain acceptable hygienic standards in relevant meat operations. There is more emphasis on slaughter hygiene in GHP schemes for slaughterhouses and more emphasis on meat processing hygiene in GHP schemes for meat products manufacturing enterprises.

Hazard Analysis and Critical Control Point Scheme (HACCP): HACCP are factory and product specific strictly sanitary control schemes that shall prevent, detect, control and/or reduce to save levels accidentally occurring hazards to consumers' health. Despite GHP in place, accidental hazards cannot be ruled out and may occur at any processing step of the individual meat product. Specifically for meat processing plants, such hazards may be provoked by failures such as batches of incoming raw meat materials with abnormal tissues or heavy contamination, breakdowns in refrigeration, failure in cooking/sterilization operations, etc.

Meat Inspection

- **Antemortem examination:** The animals to be slaughtered are first examined by a qualified veterinary surgeon; this is called antemortem examination. The diseased animal and sick animal are excluded and other healthy animal are passed for slaughter. The main causes of rejection include tuberculosis, pregnancy, diarrhea, emaciation, foot rot, etc.
- **Postmortem examination:** The examination that is carried out soon after slaughter is called postmortem examination. If any disease condition is found meat is rejected, e.g. liver fluke, cysticercus bovis, tuberculosis, etc.

11. PREVENTION OF FOOD ADULTERATION ACT (PFA),1954

Prevention of Food Adulteration Act:

Act 37 of 1954: The Prevention of Food Adulteration Bill was passed by both the house of Parliament and received the assent of the President on 29th September, 1954. It came into force on 1st June, 1955 as the Prevention of Food Adulteration Act, 1954 (37 of 1954).

List of adaptation order and amending Acts

1. The Adaptation of Laws (No. 3) Order, 1956.
2. The Prevention of Food Adulteration (Amendment) Act, 1964 (49 of 1964).
3. The Prevention of Food Adulteration (Amendment) Act, 1971 (41 of 1971).
4. The Prevention of Food Adulteration (Amendment) Act, 1976 (34 of 1976).
5. The Prevention of Food Adulteration (Amendment) Act, 1986 (70 of 1986).

Objective

- To protect the public from poisonous and harmful foods
- To prevent the sale of substandard foods
- To protect the interests of the consumers by eliminating fraudulent practices.

Meaning of Adulterant: Any material which is or could be employed for the purposes of adulteration.

Definition of Food: any article used as food or drink for human consumption other than drugs and water and includes:

- Any article which ordinarily enters into or is used in the composition or preparation of human food
- Any flavoring matter or condiments
- Any other article which the Central Government may having regard to its use, nature, substance or quality, declare, by notification in the official gazette as food for the purpose of this Act.

Concept of Adulteration

An article of food shall be deemed to be adulterated:

- If the article sold by vendor is not of the nature, substance or quality demanded by the purchaser
- If the article contains any other substance which affects the substance or quality thereof. If any inferior or cheaper substance

has been substituted wholly or in part for the article so as to affect the nature, substance or quality of the product

- If any constituent of the article has been wholly or in part extracted to affect the quality thereof
- If the article has been prepared, packed or kept under unsanitary conditions where by it has become contaminated or injurious to health
- If the article consists wholly or in part of any filthy, putrefied, rotten decomposed or diseased animal or vegetable substance or is insect-infested or is otherwise unfit for human consumption
- If the article is obtained from a diseased animal
- If the article contains any poisonous or other ingredient which renders it injurious to health
- If the container of the article is composed, whether, wholly or in part of any poisonous or deleterious substance which renders its contents injurious to health
- If any coloring matter other than that prescribed in respect thereof is present in the article or if the amounts of the prescribed coloring matter which is present in the article are not within the prescribed limits
- If the article contains any prohibited preservative or permitted preservative in excess of the prescribed limits
- If the quality or purity of the article falls below the prescribed limits of variability which renders it injurious to health
- If the quality or purity of the article falls below the prescribed standard or its constituents are present in quantities not within the prescribed limits of variability which renders it injurious to health.

Sale of Certain Admixtures Prohibited

Sale by himself or by his servant or agent is prohibited in case of:

- Cream which has not been prepared exclusively from milk or which contains less than 25% of milk fat
- Milk which contains added water
- Ghee which contains any added matter not exclusively derived from milk fat
- Selling skimmed milk as whole milk
- Mixture of two or more edible oils as an edible oil
- Vanaspati to which ghee or any other substance has been added
- Any article of food which contains any artificial sweetener beyond the prescribed limit

- Turmeric containing any foreign substance
- Mixture of coffee and other substance except chicory
- Dahi or curd not made out of milk
- Milk or milk products containing constituents other than of milk.

Procedure for Sampling and Analysis

Any food inspector can enter and inspect any place where any article of food is manufactured or stored for sale or stored for the manufacture of any other article of food for sale or exposed or exhibited for sale or where any adulterant is manufactured or kept and take samples of such article of food or adulterant for analysis.

- Notice will be issued by the inspector in writing then and there to the seller indicating his intention
- Three samples are taken and the signature of the seller is affixed to them
- One sample is sent for analysis to Public Analyst under intimation to the Local Health Authority
- The other two samples are sent to the local health authority for further reference.

Penalties

Guilt will be punished with imprisonment for a term which shall not be less than six months and up to 3 years and with fine up to one thousand rupees.

Important Miscellaneous Provisions

- If any extraneous additions of coloring matter is added, the same should be indicated on the labels
- From the labels the blending composition of ingredients should be clear to the customer
- Sale of khesari gram individually or as an admixture is prohibited
- Prohibition of use of carbide (acetylene) gas in ripening is prohibited
- Sale of ghee with Reichert value less than the permitted level
- Sale of admixture of ghee or butter is prohibited
- Addition of artificial sweetener should be mentioned on the label
- Sale of food colors without license prohibited
- Sale of insect damaged dry fruits and nuts prohibited
- Food prepared in rusted containers, chipped enamel containers

and untinned copper/brass utensils are treated as unfit for human consumption

- Containers not made of plastic material which is not according to the standards are not to be used
- Selling salseed fat or any other purpose except for bakery and confectionery is prohibited
- Store of insecticides in the same premises where food articles are stored is prohibited
- Milk powder or condensed milk can be sold only with ISI mark
- Use of more than one type of preservative is prohibited
- Crop contaminants beyond certain specified level is treated as adulterant
- Naturally occurring toxic substances in the food material beyond certain level is considered as unfit for human consumption
- No antioxidant, emulsifiers and stabilizing agent is permitted beyond the prescribed level
- No insecticides should be sprayed on the food items
- Oils can be manufactured only in factories licensed for such purpose.

SHORT ANSWER QUESTIONS

Q.1 What is sewage?

Ans. Sewage: Sewage is a water carried waste either in the form of solution or suspension that is needed to be removed from the community. Sewage contains 99.9% water and 0.1% solid matter in the form of excreta. It is characterized by volume or rate of flow, physical condition, chemical and toxic constituents and its bacteriologic status.

Q.2. List out four legislative acts regulating the environment.

Ans. The scope of environment protection is very wide. It includes many areas like forest, air, sound, soil, plant, animal kingdom, etc. Central govt. has enacted several laws, acts, rules and by laws for maintenance, safety and protection of environment. Some of these are mentioned below:

- The Water (Prevention and Control of Pollution) Act, 1974
- The Air (Prevention and Control of Pollution) Act, 1981
- The Environment (Protection) Act, 1986
- Manufacture, Storage and Import of Hazardous Chemical Rules, 1989

- The Forest (Conservation) Act, 1980
- The Wildlife Protection Act, 1972
- The Public Liability Insurance Act, 1991
- The National Environment Appellate Authority Act, 1997

Q.3. What is index case?

Ans. Index case is the initial patient in the population of an epidemiological investigation or more generally, the first case of a condition or syndrome (not necessarily contagious) to be described in the medical literature, whether or not the patient is thought to be the first person affected. It is also known as primary case or patient zero.

The **index case** is the first patient that indicates the existence of an outbreak. Earlier **cases** may be found and are labeled primary, secondary, tertiary, etc. 'Patient Zero' was used to refer to the **index case** in the spread of HIV in North America.

Q.4. List down the types of ventilation.

Ans. Types of Ventilation:

- **Natural Ventilation:** It is the use of wind and temperature differences to create airflows in and through buildings.
- **Task Ventilation:** Task or personalized ventilation is a method for providing occupants with control of a local supply of air so that they can adjust their individual thermal environment. Controlled variables could be the supply-air temperature, velocity, direction, the ratio of room air to outside in the supply air, and the radiant temperature.
- **Mechanical Ventilation:** This system supplies the required air flow at a constant rate. Ventilation is supplied by forcing air through the ducting with the use of a fan. The use of the fan however uses a lot of energy and consequently greater CO_2 emissions. There are four systems to achieve artificial ventilation: Exhaust system, Propulsion system, Balanced system and Air conditioning system.
- **Hybrid Ventilation:** Hybrid ventilation is the mix of natural and mechanical ventilation. In this project there is only one aspect of mechanical ventilation, which contributes to the hybrid one: The fan which enhances the natural stack effect if the conditions are poor.

Q.5. What is the composition of air?

Ans. Air is a mixture of gases that forms atmosphere. Average composition of gases in the atmosphere is given below:

- Oxygen: 20.96%
- Nitrogen: 78.01%
- Carbon dioxide: 0.03%
- Other than these, traces of rare gases like argon, helium, neon, xenon, etc. are also present in traces amount. These are called rare gases.

In addition to these, air also contains water vapors, traces of ammonia, and suspended matter such as bacteria, dust, spores and vegetable debris.

Q.6. Write down two noise control measures.

Ans.
- **Control at source:** This is achieved by stopping or enclosure of noise source.
- Use of Sound proof material in the building
- Use of safety devices such as ear plugs to protect the person
- Educating public regarding environment protection from noise pollution
- Determining the limit of noise and controlling the noise through law.
- Bans on horns in public places

Q.7. Enlist two milk borne diseases.

Ans. Milk Borne diseases

- Transmissible disease:
  - Salmonellosis
  - Bacillary dysentery
  - Diphtheria
  - Scarlet fever
  - Human tuberculosis
  - Cholera
  - Amebic dysentery
- Zoonotic Disease
  - Bovine tuberculosis
  - Brucellosis
  - Anthrax
  - Q fever
  - Listeriosis
  - Cow pox
  - Foot and mouth disease.

Q.8. Explain slaughter houses.

Ans. A **slaughter house** or **abattoir** is a facility where animals are slaughtered for consumption as food for humans. A place where animal are killed for their meat is termed as slaughter houses. Slaughter houses that process meat not intended for human consumption are sometimes referred to as knacker's yards or knackeries, used for animals that are not fit for consumption or can no longer work on a farm such as horses that can no longer work.

Slaughtering animals on a large scale poses significant logistical problems, animal welfare problems, and public health requirements, and public aversion in many cultures influences the location of slaughter houses.

Animal welfare and animal rights groups frequently raise concerns about the methods of transport, preparation, herding, and killing within some slaughter houses under the example of animal rights activists such as Howard Lyman and Ric O'Barry.

Q.9. Mention any two methods to remove temporary hardness of water.

Ans. Removal of Temporary Hardness: There are two methods used for the removal of temporary hardness from hard water.

1. **Boiling Method:** The temporary hardness of water is removed by simple boiling the water. In this method the calcium and magnesium bicarbonate present in water and decomposed into calcium and magnesium carbonates, which are insoluble in water, hence they settle down and soft water is drained.

   $$Ca(HCO_3)_2 \rightarrow CaCO_3\downarrow + CO_2 + H_2O$$

   $$Mg(HCO_3)_2 \rightarrow MgCO_3\downarrow + CO_2 + H_2O$$

2. **Clark's Method:** This method is used to remove hardness from water on a large scale. A calculated amount of lime water ($Ca(OH)_2$) is added to tanks containing hard water. The bicarbonates of calcium and magnesium present in water are converted into soluble carbonates which settle down at the bottom and the soft water is drained off.

   $$Ca(HCO_3)_2 + Ca(OH)_2 \rightarrow 2CaCO_3\downarrow + 2H_2O$$

   $$Mg(HCO_3)_2 + Ca(OH)_2 \rightarrow CaCO_3\downarrow MgCO_3 + 2H_2O$$

Q.10. Write any two treatment for drug poisoning.

Ans. Treatment will be dictated by the specific drug taken in the overdose. Information provided about amount, time, and underlying medical problems will be very helpful.

- The stomach may be washed out by gastric lavage (stomach pumping) to mechanically remove unabsorbed drugs from the stomach.
- Activated charcoal may be given to help bind drugs and keep them in the stomach and intestines. This reduces the amount absorbed into the blood. The drug, bound to the charcoal, is then expelled in the stool. Often, a cathartic is given with the charcoal so that the person more quickly evacuates stool from his or her bowels.
- Agitated or violent people need physical restraint and sometimes sedating medications in the emergency department until the effects of the drugs wear off. This can be disturbing for a person to experience and for family members to witness. Medical professionals go to great lengths to use only as much force and as much medication as necessary. It is important to remember that whatever the medical staff does, it is to protect the person they are treating. Sometimes the person has to be intubated (have a tube placed in the airway) so that the doctor can protect the lungs or help the person breathe during the detoxification process.
- For certain overdoses, other medicine may need to be given either to serve as an antidote to reverse the effects of what was taken or to prevent even more harm from the drug that was initially taken. The doctor will decide if treatment needs to include additional medicines.

Q.11. Explain the components of slow sand filter.

Ans. A slow sand filter consists basically of the following components:

- **Housing:** Filters can be constructed in tanks with non-reactive surfaces such as plastic or fiberglass lined galvanized tanks, poly or concrete tanks of various sizes from 205 liters up to 100,000 liter tanks.
- **Water layer:** The water layer above the filter bed provides the head to push water through the filter bed. It is convenient as a water storage zone and provides an effective temperature buffer to stabilize the filter and

protect the biological activity occurring in the top layers of filter bed.

- **Filter bed:** The filter bed consists of a uniform fine particle sand mixture as specified. The most critical design feature of the SSF is using a correct sand or alternative media. The filter bed is built to a depth of 1–1.5 m (or more) with a minimum of .8 m on smaller filters.
- **Sand specifications:** Sand is characterized by the diameter of the individual sand grains (e.g. 0.15–.35 mm) and the effective size of the composite sand, the ES or d10. d10 is defined as the sieve size in mm that permits passage of 10% by weight of the sand.
- **Drainage system:** A gravel drainage system is provided at the bottom of the filter to prevent movement of the fine sand into the filter outlet. The use of a geo-textile fabric may be considered to support the sand as an alternative to some gravel layers. The bottom layer of gravel supports perforated drainage pipes which may simply bisect the filter or in a large filter form a network of connecting pipes across the base.
- **Flow control:** A regulating tap should be connected to the filter outlet to control the flow rate. On large filters a flow meter is sometimes installed for use in monitoring the flow rate.

Q.12. Distinguish between Effluent and Sewage with two characteristics.

Ans. 1. **Definition**: Sewage may be defined as water from a community containing solid and liquid excreta (from houses, street washing, factories and industries. Whereas effluent is any liquid that has gone down a residential drain mostly containing soap, laundry discharge, water from sinks, etc.

2. **Size of the solids in liquid**: Effluent can contain solids up to ¾″ in size whereas sewage has also gone down a residential drain but can contain solids up to 2″ in diameter.

Q.13. Write four criteria for good lightening.

Ans. Appropriate lighting is essential for good eye sight and vision. Following are the criteria for good lightening.

1. **Sufficiency:** Sufficient intensity of light in the room so that it does not put strain eyes while doing activities e.g. reading or doing other work.
2. **Color and distribution of light:** Usually white light (tube light) should be used. Distribution of light should be even.
3. **Steadiness:** Light should be steady. Avoid flickering of light, color, movement of light in circles.
4. **Absence of glare:** Glare should not be there.

Q.14. Mention any four activities of sub-center.

Ans. Activities of sub-center:

- Maternal and child health:
  - Early registration of pregnant women.
  - Minimum four antenatal checkup
  - Identification of high-risk pregnancy
  - Promotion of institutional delivery
  - Postnatal health visit on 0, 3, 7 and 42nd day
  - Counseling on diet, hygiene, contraception, clean and safe delivery, etc.
- **Family planning and contraception:**
  - Provision of contraception
  - IEC (Information, education and communication) to adapt appropriate family planning methods.
- **Safe abortion services:** Counseling and appropriate referral for safe abortion services
- **Curative services:** Providing treatment for minor ailments. Appropriate and prompt referral.
- **School health services:** Staff of sub-centres provides assistance to school health services.

Q.15. List down any four sources of radiation exposure:

Ans. Sources of radiation exposure are:

- Radon and Thoron (37%)
- Industrial (<0.1%)
- Occupational (<0.1%)
- Nuclear medicine (12%)
- Computed tomography (24%)
- Terrestrial background (3%)
- Internal background (5%)
- Consumer (2%)
- Conventional radiography/fluoroscopy (5%)
- Space background (5%).

Q.16. Acts regulating food hygiene:

Ans. 1. **Prevention of Food Adulteration Act (PFA):** The Prevention of Food Adulteration Bill was passed by both the house of Parliament and received the assent of the President on 29th September, 1954. It came into force on 1st June, 1955 as the Prevention of Food Adulteration Act, 1954 (37 of 1954). It is an Act to make provision for the prevention of adulteration of food.

2. **Food Safety and Standards Act, 2006 (FSSA):** FSSA, 2006 is an Act enacted to keep with changing needs/requirements of time and to consolidate the laws relating to food and to establish the Food Safety and Standards Authority of India. The Act was needed to bring out a single statutory body for food laws, standards setting and enforcement so that there is one agency to deal and no confusion in the minds of consumers, traders, manufacturers and investors which was due to multiplicity of food laws.

3

Epidemiology

LONG ANSWER QUESTIONS

Q.1. a. Define epidemiology.
b. Explain the uses of epidemiology.
c. Discuss the different methods of epidemiology.
(2 + 3 + 10 = 15 Marks)

Q.2. a. Enlist the aims of epidemiology.
b. Explain its scope and uses of epidemiology.
c. Discuss descriptive epidemiology.(3 + 7 + 5 = 15 Marks)

SOLVED QUESTIONS PAPER

Q.1. a. Define epidemiology.
b. Explain the uses of epidemiology.
c. Discuss the different methods of epidemiology.

(A) DEFINITION OF EPIDEMIOLOGY

Epidemiology is the study of the frequency, distributions and determinants of health related sates or events in specified population and the application of this study to control health problems (Last, 1988).

The study of the distribution and determinants of disease frequency in man (Mac Mahon, 1960).

Epidemiology is that branch of medical science which deals with epidemics (Parkin, 1873).

(B) USES OF EPIDEMIOLOGY

- Study the occurrence and distribution of disease in a community
- Identify the determinants of diseases
- Diagnose the health status of a community
- Estimate the risk
- Plan effective need based health services
- Determine the effectiveness of health services planned
- Determine the usefulness and effectiveness of new/innovative techniques, measures and program.
- Complete the clinical picture of chronic diseases
- Identify syndromes by describing the distribution and association of clinical phenomenon in the population
- Forecast the likely occurrence of diseases on the basis of epidemiological principles.

(C) METHODS OF EPIDEMIOLOGY

- **Descriptive method**: It is concerned with the study of frequency and distribution of disease and health related events in population in terms of person, place and time.
  - **Personal characteristics** such as age, sex, race, marital status, occupation, education, income, social class, habits, etc.
  - **Place distribution** of cases, i.e. areas of high concentration, low concentration and spotting of cases.
  - **Time distribution**/trends, such as year, month, season, weak, day, hour of the onset of disease.

  Procedures to conduct descriptive studies:
  - Define the population to be studied
  - Defines the disease
  - Describe the disease by time, place and person
  - Measurement of disease
  - Comparing with the known indices
  - Formulation of hypothesis.
- **Analytical epidemiology:** The objective is not to formulate hypothesis; but to test hypothesis. It further divides into two parts
  1. **Experimental approach:** A hypothesis is developed and an experimental model is constructed in which one or more selected factors are manipulated. The effect of the manipulation will either confirm or disprove the hypothesis. An example is the evaluation of the effect of a new drug on

a disease. A group of people with the disease is identified, and some members are randomly selected to receive the drug. If the only difference between the two is use of the drug, the clinical differences between the groups should reflect the effectiveness of the drug.

Types:

- Randomized Control Trial (RCT)
- Field Trial
- Community Trails

2. **Observational approach:** Observational methods are more commonly applied in epidemiology as here subject is human; so limited situation can be experimented. In an observational study, the epidemiologist simply observes the exposure and disease status of each study participant. It is of three types:

   - **Prospective/cohort studies**: A cohort study is similar in concept to the experimental study. In a cohort study, the epidemiologist records whether each study participant is exposed or not, and then tracks the participants to see if they develop the disease of interest. Note that this differs from an experimental study because, in a cohort study, the investigator observes rather than determines the participants' exposure status. After a period of time, the investigator compares the disease rate in the exposed group with the disease rate in the unexposed group. The unexposed group serves as the comparison group, providing an estimate of the baseline or expected amount of disease occurrence in the community. If the disease rate is substantively different in the exposed group compared to the unexposed group, the exposure is said to be associated with illness.

     Steps:

     - Selection of study subjects
     - Obtaining data on exposure
     - Selection of comparison groups
     - Follow-up
     - Analysis.

These studies are sometimes called **follow-up** or **prospective** cohort studies, because participants are enrolled as the study begins and are then followed prospectively over time to identify occurrence of the outcomes of interest.

An alternative type of cohort study is a **retrospective** cohort study. In this type of study both the exposure and the outcomes have already occurred. Just as in a prospective cohort study, the investigator calculates and compares rates of disease in the exposed and unexposed groups. Retrospective cohort studies are commonly used in investigations of disease in groups of easily identified people such as workers at a particular factory or attendees at a wedding.

- **Case control study**: In a case-control study, investigators start by enrolling a group of people with disease (at CDC such persons are called case-patients rather than cases, because case refers to occurrence of disease, not a person). As a comparison group, the investigator then enrolls a group of people without disease (controls). Investigators then compare previous exposures between the two groups. The control group provides an estimate of the baseline or expected amount of exposure in that population. If the amount of exposure among the case group is substantially higher than the amount you would expect based on the control group, then illness is said to be associated with that exposure. The key in a case-control study is to identify an appropriate control group, comparable to the case group in most respects, in order to provide a reasonable estimate of the baseline or expected exposure.

  Steps:
  - Selection of cases and control
  - Matching
  - Measurement of exposure
  - Analysis and interpretation

  Features:
  - Both exposure and outcome has occurred before the onset of disease.
  - Study proceeds backwards from effect to cause.
  - It uses control or comparison group to support or repute an inference.

- **Cross sectional study**: In this third type of observational study, a sample of persons from a population is enrolled and their exposures and health outcomes are measured simultaneously. The cross-sectional study tends to assess the presence (prevalence) of the health outcome at that point of time without regard to duration. For example, in a cross-sectional study of diabetes, some of the enrollees with diabetes may have lived with their diabetes for many years, while others may have been recently diagnosed.

Q.2. a. Enlist the aims of epidemiology.
b. Explain its scope and uses of epidemiology.
c. Discuss descriptive epidemiology.

(A) EPIDEMIOLOGY

Epidemiology is the study of frequency, distribution and determinants of health related conditions in a population; and the application of this study to the prevention of disease and promotion of health.

Components of its definition:

- **Study**: Systematic collection, analysis and interpretation of data. Epidemiology involves collection, analysis and interpretation of health related data. Epidemiology is a science.
- **Frequency:** The number of times an event occurs. Epidemiology studies the number of times a disease occurs (How many times?) Epidemiology is a quantitative science.
- **Distribution:** Distribution of an event by person, place and time. It answers the question who, where and when? Epidemiology describes health events.
- **Determinants:** Factors the presence /absence of which affect the occurrence and level of an event. It answers the question how and why? Epidemiology analyzes health events.
- **Disease and other health related events**: The focus of epidemiology is not only on patients; it studies all health related condition. Epidemiology is a broader science.
- **Human population**: Epidemiology diagnoses and treats communities/population. Epidemiology is a basic science of public health.

- **Application**: Epidemiological studies have direct and practical application for the prevention of diseases and promotion of health. Epidemiology is an applied science.

Epidemiology has three main aims:

According to the International Epidemiological Association (IEA), epidemiology has three main aims:

1. To describe the distribution and magnitude of health and disease problems in human populations.
2. To identify the causes of diseases (also known as etiology).
3. To provide data essential for the management, evaluation and planning of services for the prevention, control and treatment of disease. Professionals who work in the area of epidemiology are known as epidemiologists.

Seven landmarks in the history of epidemiology:

1. **Hippocrates (460 BC):** Environment and human behaviors affects health
2. **John Graunt (1662):** Quantified births, deaths and diseases
3. **Lind (1747):** Scurvy could be treated with fresh fruit
4. **William Farr (1839):** Established application of vital statistics for the evaluation of health problems
5. **John Snow (1854):** Tested a hypothesis on the origin of epidemic of cholera
6. **Alexander Louis (1872):** Systematized application of numerical thinking (quantitative reasoning)
7. **Bradford Hill (1937):** Suggested criteria for establishing causation.

(B) SCOPE OF EPIDEMIOLOGY

Epidemiology is a young field with constantly expanding boundaries. The range of activities that may be at least partly epidemiologic includes determination of the health needs of populations, investigation and control of disease outbreaks, study of environmental and industrial hazards, evaluation of preventive or curative programs or treatments, and evaluation of the effectiveness and efficiency of intervention or control strategies.

There is a growing core of purely epidemiologic methodology that includes not only statistical methodology and principles of study design, but a unique way of thinking that is beyond the rote memorization of rules. The contribution of epidemiology to any study involving groups of people is being increasingly recognized and demanded.

Many tools of epidemiology are borrowed from other fields such as microbiology, immunology, medicine, statistics, demography, and medical geography.

- Originally, Epidemiology was concerned with investigation and management of epidemics of communicable diseases.
- Lately, Epidemiology was extended to endemic communicable diseases and non-communicable infectious diseases.
- Recently, Epidemiology can be applied to all diseases and other health related events.

Uses of Epidemiology

- Study the occurrence and distribution of disease in a community
- Identify the determinants of diseases
- Diagnose the health status of a community
- Estimate the risk
- Plan effective need based health services
- Determine the effectiveness of health services planned
- Determine the usefulness and effectiveness of new/innovative techniques, measures and program.
- Complete the clinical picture of chronic diseases
- Identify syndromes by describing the distribution and association of clinical phenomenon in the population.
- Forecast the likely occurrence of diseases on the basis of epidemiological principles.

(C) DESCRIPTIVE EPIDEMIOLOGY

The first stage of epidemiological studies which aims to study the advance and spread of disease or other health-related incidents in a population. It also identifies the associated characteristics for easy diagnosis and identification. It is based on person, place and time by analyzing disease patterns.

- Personal characteristics such as age, sex, race, marital status, occupation, education, income, social class, habits, etc.
- Place distribution: Areas of high concentration, low concentration and spotting of cases.
- Time distribution such as year, month, weak, day, hour of the onset of disease.

Aims

- Descriptive epidemiology is used for understanding and evaluating the trends followed by a disease and make comparisons with other ailments.

- It is also used to ensure that there is a planned implementation of services and also a measure of their effectiveness.
- Finding more data for analytical study of the issue.

There are two different designs to conduct descriptive studies in Epidemiology:

1. Cross-sectional studies
2. Longitudinal studies.

Procedure in Descriptive Studies

- You choose or define a population that you wish to study. This can be on the basis of region, sex or any other characteristics.
- Define the disease using an operational definition and measure its spread correctly.
- Analyze the distribution of disease based on various factors. For example examine the variance of disease based on
  - Age/sex and people related features
  - Time frames or
  - Geographical locations.
- Measure its impact in terms of fatality and effects.
- Compare with known cases and references.
- Formulate a hypothesis: What's a possible cause, which population is under grave danger, the various features of disease with relation to time, age, place, etc. and finally the treatment and expected outcome.

Uses

- In fields of research
- To ascertain the morbidity, mortality and other similar measurable features of a disease
- To formulate an effective hypothesis.

To create a data bank that can help in planning and organizing of preventive and curative services.

SHORT NOTES

(5 Marks)

Q.1. Epidemiological triad.

Q.2. Dynamics of disease transmission.

Q.3. Four levels of prevention.

Q.4. Difference between case control study and cohort study.

Q.5. Explain analytical epidemiology.

Q.6. Epidemiological measurements.

Q.7. Discuss descriptive epidemiology in detail.

1. EPIDEMIOLOGICAL TRIAD

A traditional model of infectious disease causation, known as the Epidemiologic Triad. The triad consists of an external **agent**, a **host** and an **environment** in which host and agent are brought together, causing the disease to occur in the host. The epidemiological triad is best represented diagrammatically. This represents the interaction between an agent, host or persons and environment or place within a specific time dimension. The epidemiological triad can be applied to non-infectious diseases where the agent could be 'unhealthy behaviors, unsafe practices, or unintended exposures to hazardous substances' (Miller, 2002, p. 64).

Agent
- Causative factors
- Risk factors
- Environmental exposures

Time
- Time characteristics
- Incubation/latency
- Length of disease process
- Trends and cycles

Host
- Person characteristics
- Group and population demographics

Environment
- Place characteristics
- Biological, physical, and psychosocial environments

- **Agent:** Agent or microbe that caused the disease (the 'WHAT' of the triangle). One of the first requirement for the occurrence of disease. It can be living or non-living. The disease agents have been classified into six broad categories:
  1. **Biological agent (microorganism):** These are infectious, generate disease and are poisonous, e.g. bacteria, virus, fungus, protozoa, etc.

2. **Nutritional agent:** Under or over nutrition, imbalance nutrients in diet, allergens, others, etc.
3. **Mechanical agent:** Injuries, fracture, etc. that develop due to frictions with machine or their parts.
4. **Physical agent:** Temperature, radiation, electricity, trauma, others.
5. **Chemical agent:** Acids, alkali, poisons, tobacco, medicine, drugs, others
6. **Social agents:** Like illiteracy, poverty, prostitution, drinking, drug abuse, etc.

- **Host:** Host or the organism harboring the disease (the 'WHO' of the triangle). Host factors are intrinsic factors that influence an individual exposure, susceptibility, or response to a causative agent. Host factors can be classified into following groups:
  - **Demographic factors:** Like individual sex, age, etc.
  - **Biological factors:** Some disease are genetics, e.g. diseases depending on the structure of genes or genetic factors
  - **Socioeconomic:** Like economic and social factors, education level, housing, marital status, etc.
  - **Lifestyle factors:** Customs and rituals, habits, nutrition, smoking, personality, etc.
- **Environment:** Environment or those external factors that affect the agent and the opportunity of exposure. It cause or allow disease transmission (the "WHERE" of the triangle). Environmental factors responsible for the causation of disease can be classified into three groups:
  - **Physical factors,** e.g. geology, climate (temperature, humidity, rain, etc.)
  - **Biological,** e.g. insects that transmit an agent
  - **Psychosocial,** e.g. crowding, sanitation, and the availability of health services.

2. DYNAMICS OF DISEASE TRANSMISSION

Dynamics of Disease Transmission involves the chain of infection. It demonstrates the process by which infectious diseases are transmitted from the reservoir to the susceptible host. **Communicable Disease is** an illness caused by an infectious agent or its toxins, which can be transmitted directly or indirectly to a well person. Communicable diseases are caused either by bacteria or virus. Sources of infection consist of man, animal, contaminated food or water, insects and environmental factors, such as dust and dirt.

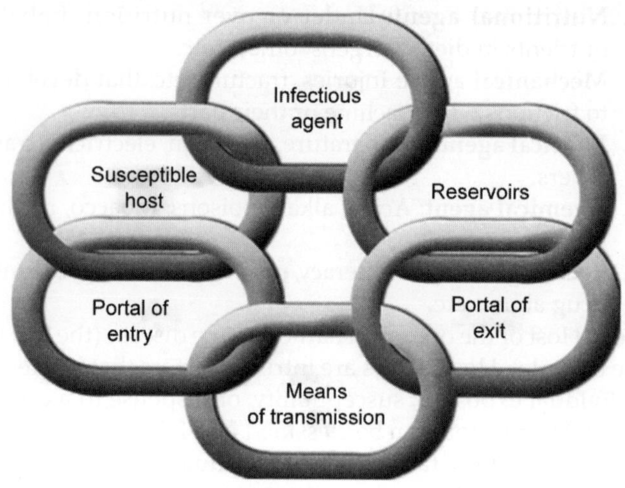

Causative/Infectious Agent

- Pathogenicity – ability to cause disease
- Virulence – (disease severity) and invasiveness (ability to enter and move through tissue)
- Infective dose – number of organisms needed to initiate infection
- Organisms specificity (host preference) antigenic variations
- Elaboration of toxin
- Viability – ability to survive outside the host
- Invasiveness – ability to penetrate the cell.

Reservoir

Natural habitant of the organism that is where resides and multiplies.

- Human – man is the reservoir of the diseases that is more dangerous to humans than to other species.
- Animal – responsible for infestations with trophozoite, worms, etc.
- Non-animal – street dust, garden soil, lint from bedding.

Carrier

Harbors the organism but without signs of infection.

Categories of Carrier

- **Incubatory**—no signs and symptoms
- **Convalescent**—disease subsided

- **Intermittent**—occasionally disseminate the infectious organism
- **Chronic**—carrying the infectious organism for years.

Mode of Transmission

It indicates the potential of the disease; conveyance of the agent to the host; it can be by common source transmission, contact source, air-borne transmission.

There are four main routes of transmission:

1. **By Contact Transmission:**
   - Direct contact (person to person)
   - Indirect contact (usually an inanimate object)
   - Droplet contact (from coughing, sneezing, or talking, or talking by an infected person)
2. **By Vehicle Route** (through contaminated items):
   - Food – salmonellosis
   - Water – shigellosis, legionellosis
   - Drugs – bacteremia resulting from infusion of a contaminated infusion product
   - Blood – hepatitis B
3. **Airborne Transmission**
   - Droplet of nuclei
   - Dust particle in the air containing the infectious agent
   - Organisms shed into environment from skin, hair, wounds or perineal area.
4. **Vector borne Transmission,** arthropods such as flies, mosquitoes, ticks and others.

Portal of Entry/Mode of Entry of Organisms into Human

- Respiratory tract
- Gastrointestinal tract
- Genitourinary tract
- Direct infections of mucous membrane/skin.

Susceptible Host

A person or animal or plant upon which parasite depends for its survival.

Host Factors:

- Age, sex, genetic
- Nutritional status, fitness, environment factors
- General physical, mental and emotional health
- Absent or abnormal immunoglobulin (Ig).

- Status of hematopoietic system, efficacy of the reticulo endothelial system (RES).
- Presence of underlying disease diabetes mellitus (DM), lymphoma, leukemia, neoplasia, granulocytopenia, or uremia.
- Patient treated with certain antimicrobials, corticosteroids, radiations, or immunosuppressive agents.

3. LEVELS OF PREVENTION

There are four levels of prevention.

1. **Primordial prevention:** This is a prevention of emergence or development of risk factors in a population group. Special attention is given to preventing chronic diseases. Main intervention is health education. In this, efforts are directed towards discouraging children from adopting harmful styles.
2. **Primary prevention:** In this, action is taken before the onset of disease. Primary preventive measures apply before a disease manifests with signs and symptoms.
   - **Health promotion**: For example, health education, environment modification, nutritional intervention, behavior change, etc.
   - **Specific protection**: For example, immunization, use of specific nutrients, chemoprophylaxis, protection against accident, carcinogens, etc.
3. **Secondary prevention:** This is aimed at patients with an existing pathology to reduce the risk of recurrence or progression. Early diagnosis and treatment are the intervention for secondary prevention. For example, all the screening test, Aspirin in arterial disease. Secondary prevention increases awareness of breast self-examination, testicular self-examination, mammography, PAP smear, BP screening, etc.
4. **Tertiary prevention:** It is aimed at avoiding further deterioration of an already existing situation. All measures to reduce or limit disability and impairment minimize suffering caused by disease process. Interventions include:
   - **Disability limitation**
   - **Rehabilitation**: Rehabilitation is restoration of an individual or a part of normal or near normal functions after disability, disease. It can be:
     - **Medical rehabilitation**: Restoration of function.
     - **Vocational rehabilitation**: Restoration of the capacity to earn a livelihood.

- **Social rehabilitation**: Restoration of family and social relation.
- **Psychological rehabilitation**: Restoration of personal dignity and confidence.

4. DIFFERENCE BETWEEN CASE CONTROL AND COHORT STUDY

S.No.	*Case Control*	*Cohort Study*
1	Proceeds from effect to cause	Proceeds from cause to effect
2	It starts with the disease	It starts with the people exposed to risk factor or suspected cause
3	Involves fewer number of subjects	Involves larger number of subjects
4	Tests whether the suspected cause occurs more frequently in those with the disease than among those without the disease	Tests whether disease occurs more frequently in exposed, than in those not similarly exposed
5	Yields relatively quick results	Requires long follow-up period
6	Suitable for the study of rare diseases	Inappropriate when the disease or exposure under investigation is rare
7	Relatively inexpensive	Expensive
8	Generally yields only estimate of relative risk	Yields incidence rate, relative risk and attributable risk
9	Cannot yield information about diseases other than that selected for study	Can yield information about more than one disease outcome

5. ANALYTICAL EPIDEMIOLOGY

This is actually the second stage of all epidemiological studies. While descriptive epidemiology deals with formulating a hypothesis through observation and study, analytical epidemiology deals with testing this hypothesis without actually indulging in experiments. Analytical epidemiology aims to research and study risk and protector factors of diseases. The key feature of analytic epidemiology is a comparison group. When investigators find that persons with a particular characteristic are more likely than those without the characteristic to contract a disease, the characteristic is said to be associated with the disease.

The characteristic may be a:

- Demographic factor such as age, race, or sex;
- Constitutional factor such as blood group or immune status;
- Behavior or act such as smoking or having eaten salsa; or
- Circumstance such as living near a toxic waste site.

There are mainly three types of analytical epidemiological studies. Let us analyse them individually:

1. Cohort study or incidence study: The main principle used here is comparing a cohort—a group having one or more similar characteristics – with another one which is similar in all manners except for one. This one will be the causative agent or the risk factor that we will be monitoring. The prospective study is usually carried out after identification of possible disease causing factors through retrospective study.

The steps involved:

- Selecting cohorts or study subjects.
- Studying exposed cohorts.
- Comparing cohorts.
- Repeating studies periodically.
- Analyzing the reports.

Example of a Cohort study is the Framingham heart study conducted by US government in the town of Massachusetts in 1948. A prospective cohort study is a longitudinal cohort study that follows over time a group of similar individuals (cohorts) who differ with respect to certain factors under study, to determine how these factors affect rates of a certain outcome. For example, one might follow a cohort of middle-aged truck drivers who vary in terms of smoking habits, to test the hypothesis that the 20-year incidence rate of lung cancer will be highest among heavy smokers, followed by moderate smokers, and then nonsmokers.

Advantages:

- Clarity of temporal sequence.
- Allow calculation of incidence.
- Facilitate study of rare exposures.
- Allow examination of multiple effects of a single exposure.
- Allows selection bias at enrollment.

2. Case control study or case reference study: Also known as retrospective study. The main principle here involved comparing two populations (one is affected by the disease and called case, the other is non-diseased and is called control) with regard to their history of exposure.

Features:

- Both exposure and outcome has occurred before the onset of disease.
- Study proceeds backwards from effect to cause.
- It uses control or comparison group to support or repute an inference.

The steps involved:

- Selecting cases
- Selecting controls with almost similar conditions
- Matching (here they are matched in all features except risk factor)
- Measure exposure
- Analysis and interpretation.

3. Cross sectional study: It is an observational study in which exposure and disease are determined at the same point in time in a given population. In terms of studies, this is the most distinct of three as it provides analysis on a population level rather than individual level. Here, the analysis is done across a cross section of population and then its results are projected to the entire population. It gives us a better 'rough idea' about some diseases but lacks the real accuracy needed at high levels. It also fails to give a time sequence and history for the disease thereby blurring the causality.

6. EPIDEMIOLOGICAL MEASUREMENTS

There are several means by which the occurrence of disease may be measured. The commonly used measures of incidence and prevalence can be distinguished by differences in the time of disease onset. **Incidence** is a count of *new cases* of the disease (or outcome). **Prevalence**, on the other hand, counts *both new and existing cases* of the disease.

Typical outcomes for an epidemiologic study, (sometimes refferred to as the 'D's of Epidemiology) are as follows:

Outcomes of Epidemiology

- Death
- Disease/Illness: Physical signs, laboratory abnormalities
- Discomfort: Symptoms (e.g. pain, nausea, dyspnea, itching, tinnitus)

- Disability: Impaired ability to do usual activities
- Dissatisfaction: Emotional reaction (e.g. sadness, anger)
- Destitution: Poverty, unemployment.

The first two, death and disease are the most commonly used.

Measures of Disease Frequency

Measures of disease frequency are used to describe how common an illness (or other health event) is with reference to the size of the population (the population at risk) and a measure of time.

Epidemiologic measures of disease frequency are of 5 types:

1. **Rate:** A fraction in which the numerator includes only individuals who meet the case definition and the denominator includes individuals in the study population who do or do not meet the case definition but could meet the case definition (at risk). A rate is dependent upon time. In other words, a proportion over a particular period of time. An epidemiologic rate will contain the following: Disease frequency (numerator), unit of population size, and the time period during which the event occurred, e.g. 44 cases of colon cancer per 100,000 population in Pennsylvania during 2000.
2. **Ratio:** A/B; a special fraction in which the numerator includes only individuals who meeting one criterion (e.g. the case definition) and the denominator includes only individuals in the study population who meet another criterion (e.g. do not meet the case definition but are at risk). A ratio is not dependent upon time. A ratio *as a measure of disease frequency* is used infrequently, in special situations (not to be confused with an odds-ratio or risk-ratio).
   Ex: 1 case of colon cancer for every 1 case of breast cancer.
   Ex: 2 female cases of major depression to 1 male case of major depression.

   The next two measures also have a time factor.
3. **Proportion**: A/(A+B); a fraction in which the numerator (A) includes only individuals who meet the case definition and the denominator totals the numbers of individuals who meet the case definition plus those in the study population who do not meet the case definition and are at risk.

   A proportion is not dependent upon time. It may be expressed as a fraction or a percentage. A proportion indicates the fraction of the population that is affected by the disease or condition. It is linked to estimating risk.

Ex: 30% of persons over 50 years of age have been screened for colon cancer:
Ex: Calculating the proportion of women with cervical cancer requires a special consideration. Cervical cancer only occurs in women with a cervix. A woman who has had a complete hysterectomy is no longer are at risk for developing cervical cancer. This is a large segment of the population of older women. The National Women's Health Information Center of the US Department of Health and Human Services reports that 1 in 3 women have had a hysterectomy by age 60. Thus, women with hysterectomies are not included in the denominator when calculating the proportion of women with cervical cancer as part of the population at risk.

4. **Risk**: The probability of an individual meeting the case definition (person-time rate). Risk is dependent upon time.
   Ex: 0.00044 colon cancer cases per person-year (typically derived from a cohort study in which each at risk person is followed over time until he/she is no longer at risk).
   Each measure serves to characterize the disease giving valuable information about contagiousness, incubation period, duration, and mortality of the disease.
5. **Count:** The number of individuals who meet the case definition;
   Ex: 9188 cases of invasive colorectal cancer in Pennsylvania in 2005 (PA Cancer Registry data)
   Calculating the magnitude of disease occurrence with a count is simple and useful for certain purposes, such as allocating health resources. For other purposes, it is more helpful to have a denominator under the count that indicates the size of the study population. The remaining four measures address this.

Other Commonly Used Measures of Disease Frequency in 'Epidemiology'

$$\text{Age/sex specific mortality rate} = \frac{\text{number of deaths in year in specific age/sex group}}{\text{mid-year population of age or sex group}} \times 1000$$

$$\text{Birth rate} = \frac{\text{number of births in a year}}{\text{mid-year population}} \times 1000$$

$$\text{Fertility rate} = \frac{\text{number of live births in year}}{\text{mid-year population of women aged 15–44}} \times 1000$$

$$\text{Infant mortality rate} = \frac{\text{number of deaths in year} < 1 \text{ year of age}}{\text{number of live births in year}} \times 1000$$

$$\text{Perinatal mortality rate} = \frac{\text{number of stillbirths + deaths} < 7 \text{ days in a year}}{\text{total number of births (live + still) in a year}} \times 1000$$

$$\text{Neonatal mortality rate} = \frac{\text{number of deaths in year} < 28 \text{ days of age}}{\text{number of live births in a year}}$$

$$\text{Case fatality rate (\%)} = \frac{\text{number of deaths in year (from specific disease)}}{\text{number of cases of that disease in a year}} \times 100$$

$$\text{Proportional mortality rate due to TB} = \frac{\text{total number of deaths due to TB}}{\text{total number of deaths due to all causes}} \times 100$$

7. DESCRIPTIVE EPIDEMIOLOGY

The first stage of epidemiological studies which aims to study the advance and spread of disease or other health-related incidents in a population. It also identifies the associated characteristics for easy diagnosis and identification. It is based on person, place and time by analyzing disease patterns.

- Personal characteristics such as age, sex, race, marital status, occupation, education, income, social class, habits, etc.
- Place distribution: Areas of high concentration, low concentration and spotting of cases.
- Time distribution such as year, month, week, day, hour of the onset of disease.

Aims

- Descriptive epidemiology is used for understanding and evaluating the trends followed by a disease and make comparisons with other ailments.

- It is also used to ensure that the there is a planned implementation of services and also a measure of their effectiveness.
- Finding more data for analytical study of the issue.

There are two different designs to conduct descriptive studies in epidemiology:

1. Cross-sectional studies
2. Longitudinal studies

Procedure in descriptive studies:

- You choose or define a population that you wish to study. This can be on the basis of region, sex or any other characteristics.
- Define the disease using an operational definition and measure its spread correctly
- Analyse the distribution of disease based on various factors. For example examine the variance of disease based on
  - Age/sex and people related features
  - Time frames or
  - Geographical locations
- Measure its impact in terms of fatality and effects.
- Compare with known cases and references
- Formulate a hypothesis: What's a possible cause, which population is under grave danger, the various features of disease with relation to time, age, place etc; and finally the treatment and expected outcome.

Uses

- In fields of research
- To ascertain the morbidity, mortality and other similar measurable features of a disease
- To formulate an effective hypothesis
- To create a data bank that can help in planning and organizing of preventive and curative services

VERY SHORT ANSWER QUESTIONS

(2 Marks)

Q.1. Explain iceberg of disease.

Ans. According to the concept of iceberg of disease, disease in a community may be compared with an iceberg. The floating tip of the iceberg represents what the physician sees in the community. The tip represents those persons who have showed symptoms of the disease and are recognized as cases (diseased persons).

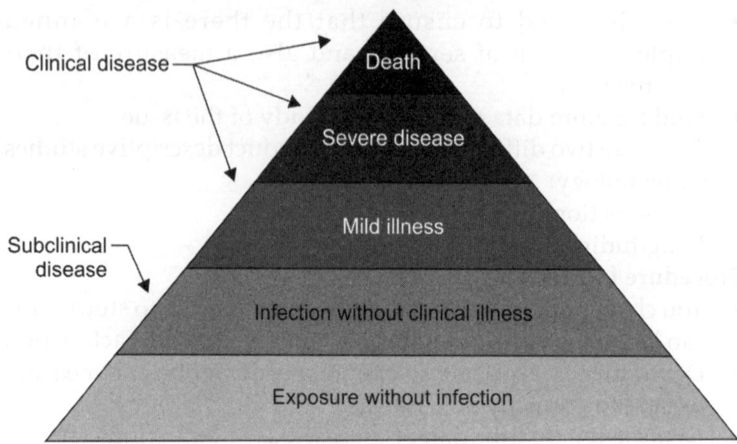

The vast submerged portion of the iceberg represents the hidden mass of the disease that is latent/presymptomatic/ undiagnosed cases and carriers in the community. The water line represents the demarcation between clinical and subclinical or undiagnosed patients.

Q.2. Define mortality.

Ans. Mortality means relative incidence of death within a particular group categorized according to age or some other factor such as occupation. **Mortality rate** or **death rate** is a measure of the number of deaths (in general, or due to a specific cause) in a particular population, scaled to the size of that population, per unit of time. Mortality rate is typically expressed in units of deaths per 1,000 individuals per year, e.g. crude death rate.

$$\text{(Crude) death rate} = \frac{\text{Total number of deaths}}{\text{Total population}} \times 1000$$

Q.3. Define endemic.

Ans. Endemic diseases are those diseases that occur regularly in an area such as Malaria in many tropical areas. In epidemiology, an infection is said to be endemic in a population when that infection is maintained in the population without the need of external inputs.

Q.4. Mention the levels of prevention.

Ans. Primary prevention is concerned with preventing the onset of disease; it aims to reduce the incidence of disease.

- **Secondary prevention** is concerned with detecting a disease in its stage, before symptoms appear and intervening to slow or stop its progression.
- **Tertiary prevention** refers to interventions designed to arrest the progress of an established disease and to control its negative consequences: To reduce disability and handicap, to minimize suffering caused by existing departures from good health, and to promote the patient's adjustment to irremediable conditions.

Q.5. Define morbidity.

Ans. Morbidity is a term used to describe how often a disease occurs in a specific area or is a term used to describe a focus on death. An example of **morbidity** is the number of people who have cancer.

Q.6. Define death rate.

Ans. The Death Rate is defined as the number of deaths per 1000 estimated mid-year population in one year. It is given by formula.

$$\text{Death rate} = \frac{\text{Number of death during the year}}{\text{Estimated mid year population}} \times 1000$$

Q.7. Classify the types of carriers.

Ans. The four types of carriers are:

1. Active Carrier.
2. Convalescent Carrier.
3. Incubatory Carrier.
4. Healthy Carrier.

Q.8. Define net reproduction rate.

Ans. The **net reproduction rate** (NRR) is the average number of daughters that would be born to a female (or a group of females) if she passed through her lifetime conforming to the age-specific **fertility** and mortality **rates** of a given year.

Q.9. Define birth rate.

Ans. The **birth rate** (technically, births/population rate) is the total number of live births per 1,000 of a population in a year. The rate of births in a population is calculated in several ways: Live births from a universal registration system for births, deaths, and marriages; population counts from a census, and estimation through specialized demographic techniques. The birth rates (along with mortality and migration rate) are used to calculate population growth.

$$\text{Birth Rate} = \frac{\text{Number of live birth during the year}}{\text{Estimated mid year population}} \times 1000$$

Q.10. Types of cohort study.

Ans. The two types of cohort study are:

1. **Prospective cohort study** (concurrent; longitudinal study): An investigator identifies the study population *at the beginning of the study* and accompanies the subjects through time.
2. **Retrospective cohort study** (historical cohort; non-concurrent prospective cohort): An investigator accesses a historical roster of all exposed and non-exposed persons and then determines their current case/non-case status.

Q.11. Two examples of naturally acquired immunity.

Ans. Active naturally acquired immunity refers to the natural exposure to an infectious agent or other antigen by the body and the body responds by making its own antibodies. Two examples of this are Measles and Chicken Pox.

Q.12. Define epidemic and give one example.

Ans. An **epidemic** is the rapid spread of infectious disease to a large number of people in a given population within a short period of time, usually two weeks or less. For example, meningococcal infections, an attack rate in excess of 15 cases per 100,000 people for two consecutive weeks is considered an epidemic.

Q.13. State two aims of epidemiology.

Ans. Two aims of Epidemiology are:

1. To describe and analyses disease occurrences and distributions in human beings.
2. To identify etiological factors in pathogenesis of diseases.

Q.14. Mention the classification of vaccine.

Ans. The classification of vaccines is as follows:

- Live attenuated vaccine
- Killed and inactivated vaccine
- Polysaccharide vaccine
- Recombinant vaccine.

Q.15. Define quarantine.

Ans. Quarantine is used to separate and restrict the movement of persons; it is a 'state of enforced isolation'. This is often used in connection to disease and illness, such as those who may possibly have been exposed to a communicable disease. Time limitation is the longest incubation period of disease. Types: Absolute, modified and segregation.

Q.16. What do you mean by mopping up?

Ans. Mopping up means to complete or put the finishing touches to a phase of particular action. In case of diseases, mopping up campaigns are door to door immunizations that are carried out in specific focal areas where the virus is known or suspected to still be circulating. Priority areas include those where polio cases have been found over the previous three years and where access to health care is difficult. Other criteria include high population density, high population mobility, poor sanitation, and low routine immunization coverage.

4

Epidemiology and Nursing Management of Common Communicable Diseases

LONG ANSWER QUESTIONS

Q.1. During home visit you have observed the problems of worm infestation in the family of Mrs. Kasuri who resides in farm house and there is no proper toilet and drainage facility. Considering above situation answer the following:

a. What are the other causative factors responsible for this problem?

b. What observations will you do regarding health habit of family members?

c. What is your plan of action regarding solving this problem?

d. What are the complications of worm infestation?

(3 + 3 + 5 + 4 = 15 Marks)

Q.2. a. List the sexually transmitted diseases.

b. Explain the responsibilities of the community health nurse in the prevention and control of HIV/AIDS.

Q.3. Define Chickenpox, clinical features and mode of its transmission. Discuss the measures for the prevention and control of chickenpox.

SOLVED QUESTIONS PAPER

Q.1. During home visit you have observed the problems of worm infestation in the family of Mrs. Kasuri who resides in farm house and there is no proper toilet and drainage facility. Considering above situation answer the following:

a. What are the other causative factors responsible for this problem?

b. What observations will you do regarding health habit of family members?

c. What is your plan of action regarding solving this problem?

d. What are the complications of worm infestation?

(A) CAUSATIVE FACTORS RESPONSIBLE FOR THIS PROBLEM

Worm infestation in children is very commonly seen in India. The common worm infestations are Threadworm, Roundworm and Hookworm. A worm is an organism, or small animal, that lives in or on and takes its nourishment from another organism.

Causative factors includes: Below are most common types of worm infections that trouble children:

- **Tapeworms:** These are flat, ribbon-like worms that can grow up to 15–30 ft and thrive in the intestine.
- **Roundworms:** They resemble earthworms and can grow up to the size of 30–35 cm.
- **Pinworms or threadworms:** As the name suggests, threadworms appear to be fine white cottony threads and live in intestine and around anus of the individual.
- **Hookworms:** These are commonly contracted through coming in touch with the contaminated soil and later enter intestine.
- Whipworm
- Ascariasis.

(B) OBSERVATIONS REGARDING THE HEALTH HABITS OF FAMILY MEMBERS

- **Coming in contact with infected surface:** The worms and their eggs are capable of surviving up to two weeks without feeding. The most common places where their kid may contact with worm infestation are:

  - Soil containing worms or eggs – in playground or outdoor play
  - Touching pets or their excrement infected with worms.
- **Inadequate handwashing:** After visiting the family, the most common and observable finding is that the family members were not washing their hands properly. It's difficult to keep young kids from putting things in their mouth. If your kid is suffering from worms, there will be itching around anus, particularly in case of pin worms. During scratching, the eggs of the worms come in contact with the skin on hand, which wherever touched tends to spread. The worse scenario is when kids put that hand back in the mouth, such as for thumb sucking or pleasure.
- **Improper hygiene:** Unwashed bedding, undergarments, filth in the room all present breeding room for worms and their eggs. Someone who has not washed hands properly can also pose a risk for others as worm eggs can stay on fingernails which can be passed to you child through touching.
- **Consuming infected food or water:** They are not washing vegetables and fruits before consumption as worm eggs can be on them. Raw or under-cooked food also carries a risk of worm infestation. Contaminated water is again a very common source of worm infestation.

  Signs and symptoms include:
  - Stomachache, weight loss or irritability.
  - Loss of appetite due to pain or discomfort
  - Anemia (especially with hookworm)
  - Nausea
  - Itching or pain around the anus, where the worms entered—this is true particularly for thread or pinworms.
  - Trouble sleeping, because of the itchiness
  - Painful or frequent urination due to urinary tract infection (UTI)
  - Blood in stool
  - Jaundice (More common in tapeworm infection).

(C) PLAN OF ACTION

- Course of antiparasitic medicine, e.g. mebendazole or albendazole, pyrantel pamoate.
- Antiworm medicines or deworming treatment should be followed.

- Diagnostic tests as prescribed by the physician
- Preventive measures includes:
  - Inculcate the habit of **frequently** and thoroughly washing the hands with a good antibacterial soap
  - It's a good idea to introduce hand sanitizer to the apple of your eyes
  - Teach them to drink clean, filtered or boiled water. Practice the same at home
  - Make sure your kids change their undergarments daily
  - Wash their bedding, pillow covers, blanket, etc. regularly
  - Sterilize your toddler's toys
  - Encourage your kid to play in dry areas and not splash in muddy puddles as these horde millions of germs
  - Make sure that the vegetables and meat are thoroughly cooked before you serve them to your family.
  - Keep your kid's nails well-trimmed. Show them how dirt collects under long fingernails and must be kept clean
  - Washing hands thoroughly before eating anything should be the rule!
  - Teach potty hygiene
  - Do not share towels and undergarments
  - Teach your kid to shower regularly. Practice thorough cleaning of private parts
  - Clean your house thoroughly and with proper disinfectants
  - Allow plenty of sunshine in your kid's room as some worms are sensitive to light.

(D) COMPLICATIONS OF WORM INFESTATION

- **Slowed growth:** Loss of appetite and poor absorption of digested foods put children with ascariasis at risk of not getting enough nutrition, which can slow growth.
- **Intestinal blockage and perforation:** In heavy ascariasis infestation, a mass of worms can block a portion of your intestine, causing severe abdominal cramping and vomiting. The blockage can even perforate the intestinal wall or appendix, causing internal bleeding (hemorrhage) or appendicitis.
- **Duct blockages:** In some cases, worms may block the narrow ducts of your liver or pancreas, causing severe pain.

Q.2. a. List the sexually transmitted diseases.
b. Explain the responsibilities of the community health nurse in the prevention and control of HIV/AIDS.

(A) SEXUALLY TRANSMITTED DISEASES

The sexually transmitted diseases are a group of communicable diseases that are transmitted by sexual contact. These are also known as venereal diseases.

The sexually transmitted diseases are listed below:

- AIDS/HIV infection
- Syphilis
- Bacterial vaginitis
- Lymphogranuloma venereum
- Genital warts
- Gonorrhea
- Trichomoniasis
- Candidiasis
- Herpes progenitalis
- Nongonococcal urethritis.

(B) RESPONSIBILITIES OF A COMMUNITY HEALTH NURSE IN THE PREVENTION AND CONTROL OF HIV/AIDS

- **Prevention of mother-to-child transmission (PMTCT) of HIV**, addressing the main mode of HIV infection in children.
- **Advise counseling and testing** (CT) for HIV, considered the gateway to comprehensive HIV prevention, care and treatment for people who test positive, as well as reinforced prevention for those who test negative.
- **Educate about male circumcision** (MC), shown to reduce the risk of female-to-male HIV transmission by 60%.
- If patient is housebound, community health nurse make coordination with the agencies that offer help specifically for HIV patients and provide home visits for services.
- Explain to the family members regarding routine household cleanliness of the bathroom, dishes, and laundry is sufficient to prevent HIV transmission.
- Explain that HIV positive family member should never share toothbrushes or razors because they can produce bleeding; a potential source of HIV transmission.

- **Prevention of medical transmission** of HIV and other infectious diseases through simple infection prevention practices, as well as postexposure prophylaxis for HIV.
- Encourage patient to disclose HIV status to their near ones; so that he/she does not feel alone. Provide emotional support to client and try to be with the client when he/she wants to share the information with the family members.
- Teach patient to optimize immune system function by sound dietary practices, exercises and regular periods of sleep.
- Provision of adult and pediatric **antiretroviral therapy** (ART), **treatment for opportunistic infections** and **palliative care**, from the facility to the community level.
- **Integration of HIV/AIDS services** with tuberculosis (TB), cervical cancer, malaria in pregnancy, family planning and maternal and child health services, to address the problem of co-infection among HIV/AIDS patients and to reach as many people as possible.
- Promote and coordinate the development of strategies, tool and guidelines to ensure rational and safe use of injections.
- Knowledge, education and literacy: HIV and stigma education drug readiness training, infection control education, e.g. positive perception of people living with HIV.
- Behavior change and communication: HIV pretest counseling, partner/couple counseling, behavior change counseling, disclosure counseling and bereavement counseling, e.g. increased uptake of HIV testing.
- Efforts should be made to reduce the fear and discrimination towards HIV infected persons in the community.
- Prevent sexual transmission of AIDS.
  - Condom promotion, provision
  - Detect and manage STI
  - Safer sex, risk reduction counseling with emphasis prevention with people living with HIV.
    - Discordant couples risk reduction
    - Continued possibility of HIV transmission on ART
    - Condom promotion and provision
    - Counsel on sexual health, return to sexuality and fertility on ART, reproductive choices
    - Counsel on substance use and risky behavior
  - Male circumcision

- Counsel the women who are HIV positive or who have an infected partner regarding avoidance of pregnancy.
- Symptomatic care should be provided to the client:
  - Diarrhea should be treated immediately to avoid dehydration.
  - Provide antiemetics as prescribed by the physician to relieve patient from nausea and vomiting.
  - Monitor vital signs: Give tepid baths or ice packs if fever persists.
  - Assess location, type, intensity of pain.
  - Encourage frequent rest periods and intermittent activity.
  - Change position 2 hours if patient is bed ridden.
  - Talk with the patient and allow him or her to express fears and concerns.

Q.3. Define Chickenpox, clinical features and mode of its transmission. Discuss the measures for the prevention and control of chickenpox.

(A) CHICKENPOX

It is also known as varicella. This is highly communicable disease in children. It occurs in both epidemic and endemic forms.

Epidemiological Factors

Etiology: Virus: Varicella Zoster Virus (VZV)
Incubation Period: 10–21 days (2–3 weeks)
Communicability period: One day before and six days after the appearance of the first vesicle.
Mode of Transmission: Droplet (direct or indirect). Dry swabs are not infectious.

Clinical Features

- Onset is sudden with **Prodromal stage**
  - Mild or light fever
  - Anorexia
  - Headache
- **Acute phase**
  - **Rash:** Successive crops of macules, papules, vesicles, crusts,(vesicles heals by forming the crusts by the end of two weeks). Different type of stages found together in this disease and this is a special character of this disease.

- Rash is itchy
- Eruptive stage remains for 4–5 days.
- The rash is centripetal in distribution, i.e. it is abundant on the trunk and scanty on the face and arms.

Treatment

- There is no specific treatment for chickenpox.
- Provide symptomatic treatment
- To relieve itching, calamine lotion should be recommended. Antihistamines, local anesthetics ointment are prescribed.
- Antibiotics for secondary infection.

Prevention and Nursing Considerations

- **Notification** of the cases to the health department
- **Isolation**
  - Using medical aseptic techniques
  - Nasal and oral discharge, clothes and linens should be disinfected
  - Keep the child in isolation until all crusts disappear.
- **Rashes**
  - Cleaning the skin according to doctor`s order once or twice daily
  - Change child`s clothes and bed linen daily to prevent skin infection
  - For itchy lesions, nails must be cut and cleaned. Mitten or gloves should be give to child so as to prevent skin scratching.
  - Observe the skin lesions for change in appearance; any change must be recorded.
  - If lesions is found in mouth; mouth wash should be recommended.
  - If lesions are there in genitals; apply cold compresses.
- For **Fever**: Check vital signs regularly
- **Disinfection** of the articles and clothing used by the patient
- Observe for the **complications** and report immediately to the doctor.
- A live attenuated varicella virus vaccine is available for the prevention of disease. Recommended for 12–18 months of age but they should not have the attack of chickenpox.

Complications: Includes abscess, encephalitis, pneumonia and glomerulonephritis may occur.

SHORT NOTES

(5 Marks)

Q.1. Control and prevention of tuberculosis

Q.2. Rabies

Q.3. Prevention and control of dengue

Q.4. Poliomyelitis

Q.5. Food borne diseases.

Q.6. Cold chain

Q.7. Zoonotic diseases

Q.8. Tetanus

Q.9. Prevention and control of malaria

Q.10. Hazards of immunization

Q.11. Immunization schedule

Q.12. Immunity

1. CONTROL AND PREVENTION OF TUBERCULOSIS

Prevention and Control of Transmission of *M. Tuberculosis*

Current recommendations for the prevention of health care associated transmission of *M. tuberculosis* involve a hierarchical approach to infection prevention and control measures, including the following:

- **Administrative controls**: For example, early case finding; institutional policies or measures that aim to reduce the time between the arrival of people with respiratory TB disease at a health care facility, diagnosis of their condition and placement in an airborne infection isolation room (AIIR).
- **Chemotherapy**: The objective of chemotherapy is to achieve bacterial cure rapidly. Current chemotherapy is based on multiple drugs with the addition of rifampicin and pyrazinamide to convectional drugs (streptomycin and Isoniazid).

Table 4.1: Treatment regimen in DOTS (directly observed treatment, short-course) chemotherapy

Category	Type of patient	Drug regimen and duration
Category I (Red Box)	• New sputum smear positive • Seriously ill sputum smear negative • Seriously ill extra pulmonary	$2(HRZE)_3 + 4(HR)_3$ For 6 months

Contd...

Contd...

Category	Type of patient	Drug regimen and duration
Category II (Blue Box)	• Sputum smear—positive relapse • Sputum smear—positive failure • Sputum smear—treatment after default	$2(HRZE)_3$ + $1(HRZE)_3$ + $5(HRE)_3$ For 8 months
Category III (Green Box)	• Sputum smear negative not seriously ill • Extrapulmonary not seriously ill	$2(HRZ)_3$ + $4(HR)_3$ For 6 months

All the drugs are administered thrice weekly. The number before the letter represents the number of months of treatment. Abbreviations are as follows: R-Rifampicin, E-Ethambutol, H-Isoniazid, S-Streptomycin, and Z-Pyrazinamide.

Daily dose regimen:

- Isoniazid : 300 mg
- Rifampicin : 450–600 mg
- Pyrazinamide : 1–1.5 gm
- Ethambutol : 800 mg
- Streptomycin : 150 mg

- **BCG Vaccination**: BCG vaccination provides protection against tuberculosis is about 80%.
- **Environmental (engineering) controls**: Environmental measures to reduce the likelihood of exposure of HCWs, other patients and visitors to viable airborne *M. tuberculosis*. These include mechanical ventilation systems (to supply clean air) in patient care areas, use of ultraviolet germicidal irradiation (UVGI) and high-efficiency particulate air (HEPA) filters.
- **Personal protection controls**: Measures directed to individual HCWs either to prevent infection (such as use of respirators) or to prevent disease if infected (such as detection and treatment of LTBI).
- **Health education:** Health education program should be directed to motivating patients for undergoing regular treatment and follow-up, disposal of sputum and cooperation with agencies organizing the program.

2. RABIES

Rabies is an acute viral disease that causes fatal encephalomyelitis in virtually all the warm-blooded animals including man. The virus is found in wild and some domestic animals, and is transmitted to other animals and to humans through their saliva (following bites, scratches, licks on broken skin and mucous membrane). Also known as hydrophobia.

Etiological Agents

- **Agent:** Lyssavirus Type-I
- **Source of infection:** Scratches or bites of infected animal
- **Incubation period:** 1 to 3 months; The time period between contracting the disease and the start of symptoms is usually one to three months; however, this time period can vary from less than one week to more than one year. The time is dependent on the distance the virus must travel to reach the central nervous system.

Signs and Symptoms

- Early symptoms can include fever, headache, malaise, pain and tingling at the site of exposure.
- These symptoms are followed by one or more of the following symptoms:
  - Violent movements.
  - Uncontrolled excitement.
  - Fear of water.
  - An inability to move parts of the body.
  - Confusion.
  - Loss of consciousness.

Once symptoms appear, the result is nearly always death.

Prevention of Human Rabies

- **Management of animal bite wound:** Washing bites and scratches for 15 minutes with soap and water, povidone iodine, or detergent may reduce the number of viral articles and may be somewhat effective at preventing transmission.
- **Antibiotic medicine and anti-tetanus** measures are to be taken.
- **Observe the animal for 10 days**: If the biting animal dies within 10 days after the bite or shows signs of illness; anti-rabies treatment should be started immediately.
- Passive immunization with Rabies Immunoglobulin (RIG).
- **Active immunization with anti rabies vaccine (ARV):** Active immunization is achieved by administration of safe and potent cell culture vaccines (CCVs) or purified duck embryo vaccine (PDEV).
- **Guide for the prophylaxis of Rabies:**
  Preprophylaxis: Preprophylaxis schedule for rabies is 3 inoculations of 1 mL given at 0, 7, 28 day.

Postprophylaxis is 5 inoculations by cell culture vaccine at 0, 3, 7, 14, 28 days and booster at 90 days (optional). The indication for postexposure vaccination with or without rabies immune globulin depends on the type of contact with the rabid animal.

Types of contact are:

- **Category I**–Touching or feeding animals, licks on the skin (No treatment is required)
- **Category II**–Nibbling of uncovered skin, minor scratches or abrasions without bleeding, licks on broken skin (Immediate vaccination)
- **Category III**–Single or multiple transdermal bites or scratches, contamination of mucous membrane with saliva from licks; exposure to bat bites or scratches. (Immediate vaccination and administration of rabies immune globulin are recommended in addition to immediate washing and flushing of all bite wounds and scratches).

- **Currently available human rabies immunoglobulin in India:** Berirab-P, Imogamrab, Plasmarab, etc.
- **Currently available anti-rabies vaccines in India:** Abhayrab, Indirab, Rabipur, Rabivax, Vaxirab, etc.

3. PREVENTION AND CONTROL OF DENGUE

Dengue is a viral disease. It is transmitted by the infective bite of *Aedes Aegypti* mosquito. Man develops disease after 5–6 days of being bitten by an infective mosquito. It occurs in two forms: Dengue Fever and Dengue Hemorrhagic Fever (DHF).

Signs and Symptoms of Dengue Fever

- Abrupt onset of high fever
- Severe frontal headache
- Pain behind the eyes which worsens with eye movement
- Muscle and joint pains
- Loss of sense of taste and appetite
- Measles-like rash over chest and upper limbs
- Nausea and vomiting.

Signs and Symptoms of DHF and Shock Syndrome

- Symptoms similar to dengue fever
- Severe continuous stomach pains
- Skin becomes pale, cold or clammy
- Bleeding from nose, mouth and gums and skin rashes
- Frequent vomiting with or without blood

- Sleepiness and restlessness
- Patient feels thirsty and mouth becomes dry
- Rapid weak pulse
- Difficulty in breathing.

Treatment of Dengue and DHF

- Prevention is better than cure
- No drug or vaccine is available for the treatment of Dengue/DHF
- The control of *Aedes Aegypti* mosquito is the only method of choice
- With early detection and proper case management and symptomatic treatment, mortality can be reduced substantially.

Vector Control Measures

Personal Prophylactic Measures

- Use of mosquito repellent creams, liquids, coils, mats, etc.
- Wearing of full sleeve shirts and full pants with socks
- Use of bed nets for sleeping infants and young children during day time to prevent mosquito bite.

Biological Control

- Use of larvivorous fishes in ornamental tanks, fountains, etc.
- Use of biocides.

Chemical Control

- Use of chemical larvicides like abate in big breeding containers
- Aerosol space spray during day time.

Environmental Management and Source Reduction Methods

- Detection and elimination of mosquito breeding sources
- Management of roof tops, porticos and sunshades
- Proper covering of stored water
- Reliable water supply
- Observation of weekly dry day.

Health Education

- Impart knowledge to common people regarding the disease and vector through various media sources like TV, Radio, Cinema slides, etc.

Community Participation

- Sensitizing and involving the community for detection of *Aedes* breeding places and their elimination.

Management of Dengue Case

- Early reporting of the suspected dengue fever
- Management of dengue fever is symptomatic and supportive
- In dengue shock syndrome, the following treatment is recommended:
  - Replacement of plasma losses
  - Correction of electrolyte and metabolic disturbances
  - Blood transfusion

(Source: NVBDCP)

4. POLIOMYELITIS

Poliomyelitis is a highly infectious disease caused by any one of the 3 Poliovirus, i.e.

a. Type 1 (Brunhilde)
b. Type 2 (Lansing)
c. Type 3 (Leon).

It attacks the brainstem and spinal cord.

Incubational Period: 7–14 days.

Communicability Period: Latter period of incubational period till the first week of acute illness.

Mode of Transmission: Oral contamination by intestinal and pharyngeal secretions of infected person.

Clinical Manifestations

- **Inapparent Poliomyelitis:** (Silent) No signs or symptoms appears.
- **Abortive Poliomyelitis:** Initial symptoms of upper respiratory tract infection: Fever, headache, vomiting, etc.
- **Non-Paralytic Poliomyelitis:** Problems as those of Aseptic Meningitis Syndrome:
  - Stiffness of neck, back and limbs.
  - Nausea and vomiting become more severe than stage II.
  - Fever.
  - Increase protein in CSF.
- **Paralytic Poliomyelitis:** This may begin with manifestations of the abortive or non-paralytic type.
  - **Spinal**: paralysis appear within a day or two after the above manifestations and 2–5 days from onset of the disease: Paralysis of limbs is the most common affected muscles, Muscles of the chest, abdominal wall, diaphragm, urinary

bladder and bowel can be affected constipation or stool incontinent and urinary incontinent may occur.
- **Bulbar:** More life-threatening. It causes damage to cranial nerve nuclei, vital centers of respiration, circulation and temperature control. It may leads to swallowing problem and regurgitation of fluids from nose and inability to swallow saliva, which puddles in the pharynx. If not aspirated chocking may occur.
- **Encephalitis:** Manifesting as encephalitis, only diagnosed as polioencephalitis if spinal or bulbar affections or both are present: Convulsion, personality disturbances.

Management

- Symptomatic treatment.
- Isolation and bed rest.
- In acute stage:
  - Put the child under close observation.
  - Notify the doctor about the degree and progress of the paralysis (7 or 8 days of the disease).
  - Rate and type of respiration and signs of respiratory distress must be observed and reported.
  - Oxygen therapy or place the child on respirator when cyanosis occurs.
  - If tracheostomy is done in case of diaphragmatic paralysis, care of tracheostomy.
- For paralysis:
  - Change position frequently. Careful positioning for affected limbs each time he is turned or moved.
  - To minimize the degree of deformity, correct body alignment and optimum position must be maintained.
  - Place the child on firm mattress.
  - Use footboard to prevent foot drop when child is on back. If the child is on abdomen, pull the mattress away from foot of bed and letting feet protrude over the edge to prevent pressure on toes.
  - Application of heat to affected muscles to relax them.
- Suction of the pharynx and postural drainage to prevent aspiration of secretions.
- For swallowing difficulties
  - Soft diet if they can swallow with difficulty.
  - If swallowing is difficult, use gavage feeding.

- **For incontinent:** Skin care and perineal region is padded to provide absorption for excretions. Catheter may be done.
- **For constipation:** Use enemas.
- Treat fever and headache.

Prevention

- **Active immunization: Trivalent oral poliovirus vaccine** (TOPV).
  - **Sabine:** Attenuated virus, which is administered orally.
  - **Salk:** Killed virus, which is administered by injection.
- **Passive immunization:** Gamma-globulin.
- If a child is affected by poliomyelitis, he must receive the vaccine to prevent further infection from the other poliovirus types.

5. FOOD BORNE DISEASES

Infectious diseases spread through food or beverages are a common, distressing, and sometimes life-threatening problem for millions of people in the United States and around the world. There are more than 250 known foodborne diseases. They can be caused by bacteria, viruses, or parasites. Natural and manufactured chemicals in food products also can make people sick. Some diseases are caused by toxins from the disease-causing microbe, others by the human body's reactions to the microbe itself.

Types of Food Borne Diseases

- **Botulism:** Botulism is a serious illness that causes flaccid paralysis of muscles. It is caused by a neurotoxin, generically called botulinum toxin, produced by the bacterium *Clostridium botulinum.*
- **Campylobacteriosis:** *Campylobacter* are a group of germs (bacteria) that are a common cause of food poisoning. Typically, food poisoning causes gastroenteritis, an infection of the gut (intestines), leading to diarrhea and often being sick (vomiting) too. Campylobacter bacteria are commonly found in raw meat, particularly poultry.
- **Hepatitis A:** Hepatitis A is a liver disease caused by the hepatitis A virus. The virus is primarily spread when an uninfected (and unvaccinated) person ingests food or water that is contaminated with the feces of an infected person. The disease is closely associated with unsafe water or food, inadequate sanitation and poor personal hygiene.

- **Norovirus Infection:** Norovirus is a very contagious virus that can infect anyone. You can get it from an infected person, contaminated food or water, or by touching contaminated surfaces. The virus causes your stomach or intestines or both to get inflamed. This leads you to have stomach pain, nausea, and diarrhea and to throw up.
- **Salmonellosis:** Salmonellosis is an infection caused by *Salmonella* bacteria. Most people infected with *Salmonella* develop diarrhea, fever, vomiting, and abdominal cramps 12 to 72 hours after infection. In most cases, the illness lasts 4 to 7 days, and most people recover without treatment.
- **Shigellosis:** Shigellosis is an infectious disease caused by a group of bacteria called Shigella. Most who are infected with *Shigella* develop diarrhea, fever, and stomach cramps starting a day or two after they are exposed to the bacteria. Shigellosis usually resolves in 5 to 7 days.

6. COLD CHAIN

'Cold Chain' refers to the process used to maintain optimal conditions during the transport, storage, and handling of vaccines and biologics, starting at the manufacturer and ending with the administration to the patient or client.

A **cold chain** is a temperature-controlled supply chain. An unbroken cold chain is an uninterrupted series of storage and distribution activities which maintain a given temperature range. It is used to help extend and ensure the shelf life of products such as fresh agricultural produce, seafood, frozen food, photographic film, chemicals, and pharmaceutical drugs. Such products, during transport and when in transient storage, are called **cool cargo**. Unlike other goods or merchandise, cold chain goods are perishable and always en route towards end use or destination, even when held temporarily in cold stores and hence commonly referred to as cargo during its entire logistics cycle. There are three basic elements needed to ensure that vaccines and biologics are handled properly:

- Well trained staff
- The right equipment
- Standard operating procedures or guidelines

Storage issues can occur as a result of malfunctioning equipment or human error.

Vaccines and biologics are sensitive. Their potency and effectiveness may be negatively impacted if they are exposed to:

- Freezing temperatures
- Heat
- Direct sunlight or fluorescent light.

Equipment for Transport to Off-site Clinics

- Insulated containers (Coolers)
  - Hard-sided insulated containers (with insulation of 30 mm to 80 mm thick) or newer Styrofoam coolers with at least two (2) inch thick walls.
  - Large enough to store vaccines and biologics, insulating materials, and icepacks during transport.
  - Tight-fitting lid and strong handles for carrying and/or wheels.
- Ice Packs
  - Keep enough ice packs frozen.
  - Do not place in direct contact with product as product(s) may freeze; place insulating materials and fillers, if required, between ice packs and product.
- Insulating Materials
  - Flexible insulating blankets, gel packs, shredded paper, cardboard, bubble wrap, or styrofoam.
  - Flexible insulating blankets or gel packs conditioned to fridge temperatures can be used to wrap around the vaccines and biologics during transport.
- Temperature Monitors
  - The use of a min/max thermometer or data logger is recommended for monitoring temperature inside the cooler during all off site clinics
  - The temperature monitor should be placed next to the products and should not come into contact with the frozen packs.

Importance of Cold Chain

- Obtaining the vaccine from the manufacturers
- Storing and transporting the vaccines
- It is used to help extend and ensure the shelf life of products
- Maintaining the supply of vaccine.
- Protecting the vaccine from sunlight.
- Keeping the vaccine at a temperature suggested by manufacture.

- Stickers (known as Viral Vaccine Monitors, or VVMs) will change color if the vaccine reaches a temperature outside of the accepted safe range of 2–8 °C.

Cold chains are common in the food and pharmaceutical industries and also in some chemical shipments. One common temperature range for a cold chain in pharmaceutical industries is 2 to 8 °C (36 to 46 °F). But the specific temperature (and time at temperature) tolerances depend on the actual product being shipped. Unique to fresh produce cargoes, the cold chain requires to additionally maintain product specific environment parameters which include air quality levels (carbon dioxide, oxygen, humidity and others), which makes this the most complicated cold chain to operate.

This is important in the supply of vaccines to distant clinics in hot climates served by poorly developed transport networks. Disruption of a cold chain due to war may produce consequences similar to the smallpox outbreaks in the Philippines during the Spanish–American War.

There have been numerous events where vaccines have been shipped to third world countries with little to no cold chain infrastructure (Sub-Sahara Africa) where the vaccines were inactivated due to excess exposure to heat. Patients that thought they were being immunized, in reality were put at greater risk due to the inactivated vaccines they received. Thus great attention is now being paid to the entire cold chain distribution process to ensure that simple diseases can eventually be eradicated from society.

The cold chain distribution process is an extension of the good manufacturing practice (GMP) environment that all drugs and biological products are required to adhere to, enforced by the various health regulatory bodies.

7. ZOONOTIC DISEASES

A zoonotic disease is a disease that can be spread between animals and humans. Zoonotic diseases can be caused by viruses, bacteria, parasites, and fungi. These diseases are very common. Scientists estimate that more than 6 out of every 10 infectious diseases in humans are spread from animals.

Any disease or infection that is naturally transmissible from vertebrate animals to humans and vice-versa is classified as a zoonosis according to the PAHO publication 'Zoonoses and communicable diseases common to man and animals'. Zoonoses have been recognized for many centuries, and over 200 have been described. They are caused by all types of pathogenic agents, including bacteria, parasites, fungi, and viruses.

Many people interact with animals in their daily lives. We raise animals for food and keep them in our homes as pets. We might come into close contact with animals at a county fair or petting zoo or encounter wildlife when we clear wooded land for new construction.

Because of these interactions, it's important to be aware of the different ways people can get zoonotic diseases.

Some examples of zoonoses, classified according to the type of causative agent, are given hereafter.

- **Viral:** For example, Rabies, Yellow fever, Japanese encephalitis, Kyasanur Forest disease, etc.
- **Bacterial:** For example, Plague, Brucellosis, Anthrax, Leptospirosis, etc.
- **Parasitic:** For example, Teniasis, Hydatid disease, Leishmaniasis, trematodosis, toxoplasmosis, etc.
- Rickettsial disease
- **Fungi:** For example, Dermatophytoses, sporotrichosis, etc.

Mode of Disease Transmission

- Coming into contact with the saliva, blood, urine, or feces of an infected animal
- Being bitten by a tick or mosquito (often called a 'vector')
- Eating or drinking something unsafe (such as unpasteurized milk, undercooked meat, or unwashed fruits and vegetables that are contaminated with feces from an infected animal).

Preventive Measures

- **Good personal hygiene:** Wash hands after handling animals and before preparing or eating food or smoking cigarettes. Unwashed hands should not be put in the mouth, including someone else's mouth.
- **Hygienic food preparation:** Food-borne diseases can be largely avoided through correct processing and hygienic food preparation.
- **Vaccination for people:** Vaccines are available for some zoonoses and they should be made use of. Abattoir workers,

farmers and vets should seek advice on Q fever vaccination. To protect against Australian bat lyssavirus, bat carers are advised to have a rabies vaccination.

- **Personal protection:** Gloves, boots and aprons or overalls should be worn when handling animals. Cover cuts and scratches with waterproof plasters. For some diseases that may be fatal to people, e.g. Hendra virus, full protective clothing is essential including respiratory protection.
- **Maintain animal health:** Farm biosecurity and animal health programs, including the use of vaccines, play an important role in reducing the risk of some zoonotic diseases. Pet owners should make sure their animals are healthy and regularly wormed; private veterinarians can provide advice on treatments.
- **Care when pregnant:** To reduce the risk of toxoplasmosis, pregnant women should not empty cat litter boxes and or handle pregnant ewes.
- **Care when immunosuppressed:** People with depressed immunity whether due to illness or medical treatments, should avoid all exposure to zoonotic diseases.
- **Suspect and stray animals:** Animals that appear ill, or carry skin infections should not be handled without taking precautions. It is also wise to avoid handling stray animals.
- **Control of pest animals:** Animals such as rats or feral pigs can carry zoonotic diseases and control programs will reduce the likelihood of transmission to people.

8. TETANUS

Tetanus, also known as **lockjaw**, is an infection characterized by muscle spasms. In the most common type, the spasms begin in the jaw and then progress to the rest of the body. These spasms usually last a few minutes each time and occur frequently for three to four weeks. Spasms may be so severe that bone fractures may occur.

Epidemiological Factors

Etiology: *Clostridium tetani* (tetanus bacillus).
Incubational Period: 3–21 days.
Communicability Period: Not communicable from man to man, as the organism usually lives in animal's intestinal tract.
Mode of Transmission: Through a wound as organism is present in soil.

Signs and Symptoms: Onset of the disease is either gradual or acute.

- Convulsions are the first warning symptoms in children.
- Excessive irritability and restlessness.
- Difficulty in swallowing.
- Stiff neck.
- Within 24–48 hours, the muscular stiffness progress:
  - Trismus, i.e. tight jaw, inability to open the mouth.
  - Stiff arm and legs, then entire stiffness of the body.
  - Swallowing usually becomes impossible.
  - Risus sardonicus due to spasm of facial muscles.
  - Opisthotonos, i.e. backward arching of the back as a result of the dominance of the extensor muscles of the spine, head draws back.

  These ongoing tetanic spasms last about 10 seconds and occur following slightest stimuli, such as, claiming the door or bumping the bed.
- Dyspnea and cyanosis can develop.
- Fever 38.5–40 °C.
- Constipation may develop.
- Lumbar puncture reveals and increase spinal fluid pressure.

Control and Prevention

- Isolation.
- Protect the child from any stimuli (auditory or tactile stimuli), so place the child in dark, quite room and minimum handling.
- If dyspnea and cyanosis are present, give oxygen.
- For tetanic spasm:
  - Protect the child from falling.
  - The nurse must be alert for number, duration and frequency of convulsion (in relation to sedation administered).
  - Record any change in trismus or inability to swallow.
- For inability to swallow:
  - IV therapy for nutrition and fluid balance.
  - Gavage feeding may be ordered. So, the nurse must report if insertion of the tube causes convulsions.
  - Accurate intake and output chart is necessary.
  - Mouth care if he can open his mouth.
- For constipation, give enema.
- Check vital signs carefully.

- If tracheostomy is performed; care of tracheostomy.
- Nasopharyngeal suction is done frequently.
- **Treatment:**
  - Antibiotics (Penicillin).
  - Antitoxin.
  - Tranquilizers.
- **Prevention:**
  - Active immunization: DPT vaccine.
  - Passive immunization: Injection of tetanus immunoglobulin or antitoxin (a few hours after a wound occur).

9. PREVENTION AND CONTROL OF MALARIA

Malaria is caused by Plasmodium parasites. The parasites are spread to people through the bites of infected female *Anopheles* mosquitoes, called 'malaria vectors.' There are 5 parasite species that cause malaria in humans, and 2 of these species – *P. falciparum* and *P. vivax* – pose the greatest threat.

Malaria Control Strategies

- **Early case detection and prompt treatment (EDPT)**
  - EDPT is the main strategy of malaria control—radical treatment is necessary for all the cases of malaria to prevent transmission of malaria.
  - Chloroquine is the main anti-malaria drug for uncomplicated malaria.
  - Drug Distribution Centers (DDCs) and Fever Treatment Depots (FTDs) have been established in the rural areas for providing easy access to anti-malarial drugs to the community.
  - Alternative drugs for chloroquine resistant malaria are recommended as per the drug policy of malaria.
- **Vector control**
  - Chemical control
    - Use of Indoor Residual Spray (IRS) with insecticides recommended under the program
    - Use of chemical larvicides like Abate in potable water
    - Aerosol space spray during day time
    - Malathion fogging during outbreaks
  - Biological control

- Use of larvivorous fish in ornamental tanks, fountains, etc.
- Use of biocides.

- **Personal prophylactic measures** that individuals/communities can take up
  - Use of mosquito repellent creams, liquids, coils, mats, etc.
  - Screening of the houses with wire mesh
  - Use of bed nets treated with insecticide
  - Wearing clothes that cover maximum surface area of the body.
- **Community participation**
  - Sensitizing and involving the community for detection of *Anopheles* breeding places and their elimination
  - NGO schemes involving them in program strategies
  - Collaboration with CII/ASSOCHAM/FICCI
- **Environmental management and source reduction methods**
  - Source reduction, i.e. filling of the breeding places
  - Proper covering of stored water
  - Channelization of breeding source
- **Monitoring and evaluation of the program**
  Monthly Computerized Management Information System (CMIS)
  - Field visits by State National Programme Officers
  - Field visits by Malaria Research Centres and other ICMR Institutes
  - Feedback to states on field observations for correction actions.

(Source: NVBDCP)

10. HAZARDS OF IMMUNIZATION

Hazards of immunization includes:

- **Reactions inherent to inoculation:** These may be local general reactions. The local reactions may be pain, swelling, redness, tenderness and development of a small nodule or sterile abscess at the site of injection
- **Reactions due to faulty techniques:** Faulty techniques may relate to:
  - Faulty production of vaccine (e.g. inadequate inactivation of the microbe, inadequate detoxication)
  - Too much vaccine given in one dose
  - Improper immunization site or route

  - Vaccine reconstituted with incorrect diluents
  - Wrong amount of diluent used
  - Drug substituted for vaccine or diluent
  - Vaccine prepared incorrectly for use (e.g. an adsorbed vaccine not shaken properly before use)
  - Vaccine or diluent contaminated
  - Vaccine stored incorrectly
  - Contraindications ignored (e.g. a child who experienced a severe reaction after a previous dose of DPT vaccine is immunized with the same vaccine)
  - Reconstituted vaccine of one session of immunization used again at the subsequent session.
- **Reactions due to hypersensitivity:** Administration of antisera (e.g. ATS) may occasionally give rise to anaphylactic shock and serum sickness.
- **Neurological involvement:** Neuritic manifestations may be seen after the administration of serum or vaccine, e.g. postvaccinal encephalitis and encephalopathy following administration of anti-rabies and smallpox vaccines.
- **Provocative reactions:** Occasionally following immunization there may occur a disease totally unconnected with the immunizing agent (e.g. provocative polio after DPT or DT administration against diphtheria).
- **Others:** These may comprise damage to the fetus (e.g. with rubella vaccination).

11. IMMUNIZATION SCHEDULE

Immunization schedule: National immunization schedule for infants, children and pregnant women:

Vaccine	When to give	Dose	Route	Site
For pregnant women				
TT-1	Early in pregnancy	0.5 mL	Intramuscular	Upper Arm
TT-2	4 weeks after TT-1*	0.5 mL	Intramuscular	Upper Arm
TT-Booster	If received 2 TT doses in a pregnancy within last 3 yrs*	0.5 mL	Intramuscular	Upper Arm

Contd...

Contd...

Vaccine	When to give	Dose	Route	Site
For infants				
BCG	At birth or as early as possible till one year of age	0.1 mL (0.05 mL till 2 month age)	Intramuscular	Left Upper Arm
Hepatitis B	At birth or as early as possible within 24 hours	0.5 mL	Intramuscular	Anterolateral side of mid-thigh
OPV-0	At birth or as early as possible within the first 15 days	2 drops	Oral	Oral
OPV-1, 2 and 3	At 6 weeks, 10 weeks and 14 weeks	2 drops	Oral	Oral
DPT 1, 2 and 3	At 6 weeks, 10 weeks and 14 weeks	0.5 mL	Intramuscular	Anterolateral side of mid thigh
Hep B 1, 2 and 3	At weeks, 10 weeks and 14 weeks	0.5 mL	Intramuscular	Anterolateral side of mid thigh
Measles	9 completed months to 12 months.	0.5 mL	Subcutaneous	Flight upper arm
Vitamin-A (1st dose)	At 9 months with measles	1 mL (1 lakh IU)	Oral	Oral
For Children				
DPT booster	16–24 months	0.5 mL	Intramuscular	Anterolateral side of mid-thigh
Measles 2nd dose	16–24 months	0.5 mL	Subcutaneous	Right upper arm
OPV Booster	16–24 months	2 drops	Oral	Oral
Japanese Encephalitis	16–24 months	0.5 mL	Subcutaneous	Left upper arm
Vitamin-A				
(2nd to 9th dose)	16 months. Then, one dose every 6 months up to the age of 5 years.	2 mL (2 lakh IU)	Oral	Oral

Contd...

Contd...

Vaccine	When to give	Dose	Route	Site
DPT booster	5–6 years	0.5 mL	Intramuscular	Upper arm
TT	10 years and 16 years	0.5 mL	Intramuscular	Upper arm
*Give TT-2 or booster doses before 36 weeks of pregnancy. However, give these even if more than 36 weeks have passed. Give TT to a woman in labor, if she has not previously received TT.				

12. IMMUNITY

Immunity is the balanced state of having adequate biological defenses to fight infection, disease, or other unwanted biological invasion, while having adequate tolerance to avoid allergy, and autoimmune diseases. There are two types of immunity.

1. **Passive immunity:** Passive immunity is the transfer of active immunity, in the form of readymade antibodies, from one individual to another. Passive immunization is used when there is a high-risk of infection and insufficient time for the body to develop its own immune response, or to reduce the symptoms of ongoing or immunosuppressive diseases.

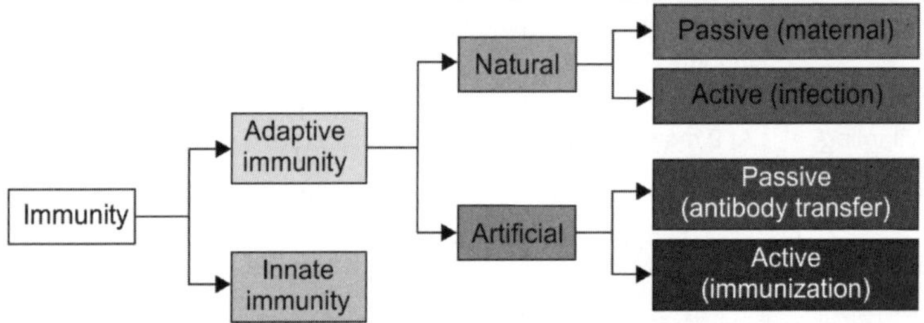

   - **Naturally acquired passive immunity:** It refers to antibody-mediated immunity conveyed to a fetus by its mother during pregnancy. Maternal antibodies (MatAb) are passed through the placenta to the fetus by an FcRn receptor on placental cells. This occurs around the third month of gestation. IgG is the only antibody isotype that can pass through the placenta. Passive immunity is also provided through the transfer of IgA antibodies found in breast milk that are transferred to the gut of the infant, protecting against bacterial infections, until the newborn can synthesize its own antibodies.

- **Artificially acquired passive immunity:** Artificially acquired passive immunity is a short-term immunization induced by the transfer of antibodies, which can be administered in several forms; as human or animal blood plasma, as pooled human immunoglobulin for intravenous (IVIG) or intramuscular (IG) use, and in the form of monoclonal antibodies (MAb). Passive transfer is used prophylactically in the case of immunodeficiency diseases, such as hypogammaglobulinemia. It is also used in the treatment of several types of acute infection, and to treat poisoning.

2. **Active immunity**: When B cells and T cells are activated by a pathogen, memory B-cells and T-cells develop, and the primary immune response results. Throughout the lifetime of an animal these memory cells will 'remember' each specific pathogen encountered, and are able to mount a strong secondary response, if the pathogen is detected again. Active immunity often involves both the cell-mediated and humoral aspects of immunity as well as input from the innate immune system.
   - **Naturally acquired active immunity:** Naturally acquired active immunity occurs when a person is exposed to a live pathogen, and develops a primary immune response, which leads to immunological memory. This type of immunity is 'natural' because it is not induced by deliberate exposure. Many disorders of immune system function can affect the formation of active immunity such as immunodeficiency (both acquired and congenital forms) and immunosuppression.
   - **Artificially acquired active immunity:** Artificially acquired active immunity can be induced by a vaccine, a substance that contains antigen. A vaccine stimulates a primary response against the antigen without causing symptoms of the disease. The term vaccination was coined by Richard Dunning, a colleague of Edward Jenner, and adapted by Louis Pasteur for his pioneering work in vaccination.

Examples of vaccines are as follows:

Bacterial vaccines

- Live: BCG vaccine for tuberculosis
- Killed vaccines: TAB vaccine for enteric fever.

Viral vaccines

- Live – sabin vaccine for poliomyelitis, MMR vaccine for measles, mumps, rubella
- Killed vaccines – salk vaccine for poliomyelitis, neural and non-neural vaccines for rabies.

  Bacterial products: Toxoids for Diphtheria and Tetanus.

VERY SHORT ANSWER QUESTIONS

(2 Marks)

Q.1. List the three complications of mumps.

Ans. The three complications associated with mumps are:

1. Viral Meningitis
2. Pancreatitis
3. Swollen testicles (orchitis) or Ovaries (ovaritis).

Q.2. List the six killer diseases.

Ans. The six killer diseases are:

1. Diphtheria
2. Polio
3. Tetanus
4. Tuberculosis
5. Measles
6. Whooping Cough.

Q.3. State the symptoms of typhoid fever.

Ans. Symptoms of Typhoid fever includes:

- A very high temperature.
- Headaches and Stomachaches
- Feeling sick
- Losing appetite
- Constipation or diarrhea.

Q.4. List the re-emerging diseases.

Ans.
1. SARS
2. Tuberculosis
3. Lyme disease
4. Influenza
5. Prion diseases.

Q.5. Mention the principles of arthropod control.

Ans. There are two major principles of control that may be employed in dealing with arthropod problems – **preventive and corrective.**

a. **Preventive control** involves the use of methods to forestall or postpone (insofar as possible) pest infestations. Generally, this type of control is more effective, more economical, permanent, and usually nonchemical in nature. It usually requires high initial expenses and results are not readily apparent.
b. **Corrective control** involves the use of methods designed to cope with existing infestations; hence, it is a 'brush fire' approach. Usually this type of control involves a low initial cost, fast results, and it is the only alternative once prevention fails. This type of control is typically less effective, more expensive in the long run, temporary in nature, and usually chemical.

Q.6. What are the cardinal features of Leprosy?

Ans. The three cardinal features/signs of leprosy are:

1. One or more hypopigmented, anesthetic skin patch (often using photos of typical lesions as a guide)
2. One or more thickened peripheral nerve.
3. A positive skin smear.

Q.7. What is the incubation period of Amebiasis?

Ans. The incubation period for *E. histolytica* infection is commonly 2–4 weeks but may range from a few days to years. The clinical spectrum of amebiasis ranges from asymptomatic infection to fulminant colitis and peritonitis to extra intestinal amebiasis, the most common form of which is amebic liver abscess.

Q.8. State any four zoonotic diseases.

Ans. The four zoonotic diseases are:

1. Tuberculosis
2. Rabies
3. Histoplasmosis
4. Leprosy.

Q.9. What is Koplik's Spot?

Ans. Koplik's spots (also Koplik's sign) are a prodromic viral enanthem of measles manifesting two to three days before the measles rash itself. They are characterized as clustered, white lesions on the buccal mucosa (opposite the lower 1st and 2nd molars) and are pathognomonic for measles.

Q.10. Name the vaccine preventable six killer diseases.

Ans. 1. Tuberculosis
2. Tetanus
3. Whooping Cough
4. Polio
5. Measles
6. Diphtheria.

Q.11. Write down the ideal time to give DPT vaccine to infants.

Ans. 6 weeks to 18 months.

Q.12. List down four Respiratory Infection.

Ans. 1. Common Cold
2. Bronchitis
3. Pneumonia
4. Sinusitis.

Q.13. What is the causative organism of Chickenpox?

Ans. The causative agent is called human herpesvirus 3 (HHV-3) or varicella zoster virus (VZV). VZV is one of eight herpesviruses known to infect humans and vertebrates. VZV only affects humans, and commonly causes chickenpox in children, teens and young adults and herpes zoster (shingles) in adults and rarely in children. VZV is known by many names, including chickenpox virus, varicella virus, zoster-virus, and human herpesvirus type 3 (HHV-3).

Q.14. State the incubation period of poliomyelitis?

Ans. For the onset of paralysis in paralytic poliomyelitis, the incubation period usually is 7 to 21 days. The response to poliovirus infection is highly variable and has been categorized on the basis of the severity of clinical presentation.

Q.15. What is Viral Hepatitis?

Ans. Viral hepatitis is liver inflammation due to a viral infection. It may present in acute (recent infection, relatively rapid onset) or chronic forms. The most common causes of viral hepatitis are the five unrelated hepatotropic viruses: Hepatitis A, Hepatitis B, Hepatitis C, Hepatitis D and Hepatitis E. In addition to the nominal hepatitis viruses, other viruses that can also cause liver inflammation include Cytomegalovirus, Epstein–Barr virus, and Yellow fever.

Q.16. What are the contraindications of OPV?

Ans. In rare instances, administration of OPV has been associated with paralytic poliomyelitis in healthy recipients and their contacts. Very rarely, OPV has caused fatal paralytic poliomyelitis in immune-compromised persons. Because OPV contains trace amounts of streptomycin, bacitracin, and neomycin, its use is contraindicated in persons who have previously had an anaphylactic reaction to OPV or to these antibiotics.

Q.17. Name any four viruses that cause diarrhea.

Ans. Many viruses cause diarrhea, including rotavirus, norovirus, cytomegalovirus, herpes simplex virus, and viral hepatitis. Infection with the rotavirus is the most common cause of acute diarrhea in children. Rotavirus diarrhea usually resolves in 3 to 7 days but can cause problems digesting lactose for up to a month or longer.

Q.18. What are the types of food poisoning?

Ans. Eight types of food poisoning are:

1. Campylobacter enteritis
2. Cholera
3. *E. coli* Enteritis
4. Ciguatera (Fish Poisoning)
5. *Listeria*
6. *Staphylococcus*
7. *Salmonella*
8. Shigellosis

Q.19. What is the mode of transformation in Amebiasis?

Ans. Amebiasis is usually transmitted by the fecal-oral route, but it can also be transmitted indirectly through contact with dirty hands or objects as well as by anal-oral contact. Infection is spread through ingestion of the cyst form of the parasite, a semi-dormant and hardy structure found in feces. Any non-encysted amebae, or trophozoites, die quickly after leaving the body but may also be present in stool: These are rarely the source of new infections. Since amebiasis is transmitted through contaminated food and water, it is often endemic in regions of the world with limited modern sanitation systems, including México, Central America, Western South America, South Asia and Western and Southern Africa.

Q.20. Define Swine Flu.

Ans. Swine flu is a respiratory illness of pigs caused by infection with swine influenza A virus (SIV). While swine flu viruses normally do not infect humans, occasional infections of humans do occur. Human cases of swine influenza A virus infection occur in individuals who have had a history of recent direct contact with pigs or close (within 6 feet) contact with pigs. Rare instances of human-to-human transmission have been documented. Swine flu infections have also occurred in individuals with no history of exposure to pigs. Symptoms typically range from a mild respiratory illness to flu-like symptoms with fever. Treatment involves the use of antiviral medications begun as soon as possible after the onset of symptoms. Vaccines are available to be given to pigs to prevent swine flu in these animals.

Q.21. Define emerging and re-emerging diseases.

Ans. Emerging infectious diseases (EIDs) are diseases of infectious origin whose incidence in humans has increased within the recent past or threatens to increase in the near future. These include new, previously undefined diseases as well as old diseases with new features. Two examples are Influenza and Lyme disease.

Re-emerging infectious diseases are diseases that once were major health problems globally or in a particular country, and then declined dramatically, but are again becoming health problems for a significant proportion of the population. Two examples are Malaria and Tuberculosis.

Q.22. What are the six 'F' in typhoid transmission?

Ans. The 6 F's in typhoid transmission are:

1. Fluids
2. Food
3. Flies
4. Fingers
5. Fomites
6. Feces.

Q.23. Name the bacterial drug given for Tuberculosis.

Ans. Active tuberculosis, particularly if it's a drug-resistant strain, will require several drugs at once. The most common medications used to treat tuberculosis include:

1. Isoniazid.
2. Rifampin (Rifadin, Rimactane)
3. Ethambutol (Myambutol)
4. Pyrazinamide.

Q.24. Name the nematodes causing hookworm infection in man.

Ans. Human hookworm disease is a common helminth infection that is predominantly caused by the nematode parasites *Necator americanus* and *Ancylostoma duodenale*; organisms that play a lesser role include *Ancylostoma ceylanicum*, *Ancylostoma braziliense*, and *Ancylostoma caninum*.

Q.25. List four drugs used in anti-retroviral treatment.

Ans.
1. Nucleoside Reverse Transcriptase Inhibitors (NRTIs): Abacavir
2. Non-Nucleoside Reverse Transcriptase Inhibitors (NNRTIs): Efavirenz
3. Protease Inhibitors (PIs): Atazanavir
4. Fusin Inhibitors: Enfuvirtide.

Q.26. List the medical treatment of Plaque.

Ans. The five drugs used as treatment includes:
1. Kenalog Injection.
2. Triamcinolone Acetonide Topical.
3. Cobetasol Topical.
4. Betamethasone Valerate Topical.
5. Aristospan Intralesional Injection

Topical treatments for psoriasis include salicylic acid. Some doctors recommend salicylic acid ointment, which smoothes the skin by promoting the shedding of psoriatic scales. Using salicylic acid over large areas of skin, however, may cause the body to absorb too much of the medication, leading to side effects.

5

Epidemiology and Nursing Management of Common Noncommunicable Diseases

LONG ANSWER QUESTIONS

Q.1. a. Define malnutrition. (2 Marks)

b. Enumerate the causes of malnutrition. (3 Marks)

c. Explain in detail about the measures to control malnutrition. (10 Marks)

Q.2. a. Define anemia. (2 Marks)

b. Enumerate the causes of anemia. (3 Marks)

c. Explain in detail about the measures to control anemia. (10 Marks)

SOLVED QUESTION PAPERS

Q.1. a. Define malnutrition. (2)

b. Enumerate the causes of malnutrition. (3)

c. Explain in detail about the measures to control malnutrition. (10)

(A) MALNUTRITION

The World Health Organization (WHO) defines malnutrition as 'the cellular imbalance between the supply of nutrients and energy and the body's demand for them to ensure growth, maintenance, and specific functions.' The term protein-energy malnutrition (PEM) applies to a group of related disorders that include marasmus, kwashiorkor (see the images below), and intermediate states of marasmus-kwashiorkor.

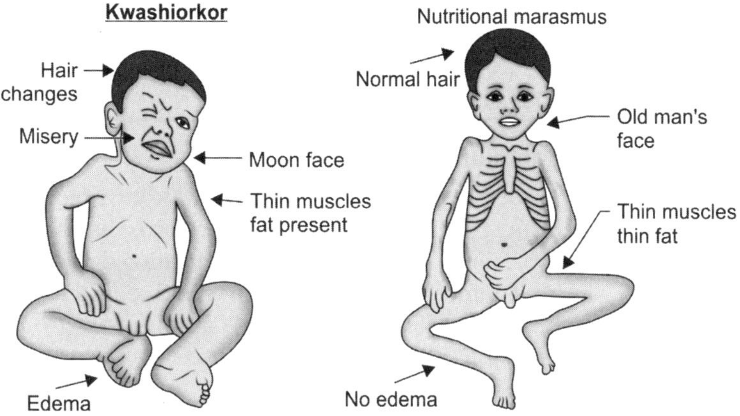

(B) CAUSES OF MALNUTRITION

- **Direct Causes:** These include:
  - **Inadequate food intake:** Inadequate food intake is the result of limited access to food in terms of quality and quantity.
  - **Diseases:** Diseases notably malaria and measles lead to loss of appetite, increased rate of metabolism due to fevers thereby increasing the body's nutrient demands. Diarrhea reduces the absorption of food nutrients, whereas vomiting decreases food intake. Intestinal parasites compete for nutrients with the body, e.g. hookworm competes for iron.
- **Indirect causes:** The most common indirect causes (social, economic, biological and environmental factors) of PEM include:
  - Food insecurity and limited access to food stuff
  - Poor water or insanitation and inadequate health services
  - Inadequate maternal and child care practices.
  - Unhealthy environment
  - Large family size
  - Improper breastfeeding and giving excessive diluted milk to children
  - Bad nutritional practices
  - Improper complementary feeding
  - Lack of health education
  - Familial disharmony.

- **Role of free radicle and alfatoxin:** Two new theories have been postulated recently to explain the pathogenesis of kwashiorkor. These include Free Radical Damage and Aflatoxin poisoning. These may damage liver cells giving rise to kwashiorkor.

(C) MEASURES TO CONTROL MALNUTRITION

Protein-energy Malnutrition

It is a group of body depletion disorders which include kwashiorkor, marasmus and the intermediate stages. It is also referred as protein calorie malnutrition. It is considered as primary nutritional problem in India. PEM is due to food gap between intake and requirement. The term Protein-energy Malnutrition (PEM) applies to a group of related disorders that includes marasmus, kwashiorkor, and intermediate states of marasmus-kwashiorkor.

Screening for Malnutrition

- **Height and weight:** The best way to identify children who are malnourished is to take their height and weight regularly once in a month. The growth chart or road to health chart offers a simple and inexpensive means of monitoring child health and nutritional status.
- **Mid-arm circumference:** Measure the mid-arm circumference of child between the age of 1–5 years of age. If measurement is found below 12.8 cm the child is considered malnourished.
- **Clinical and laboratory examination:** An examination of child from head to foot for the signs of malnutrition.

Different forms of Protein-energy Malnutrition (PEM):

- **Kwashiorkor:** The term kwashiorkor is taken from the Ga language of Ghana and means "the sickness of the weaning".
  - Williams first used the term in 1933, and it refers to an inadequate protein intake with reasonable caloric (energy) intake.
  - Kwashiorkor, also called wet protein-energy malnutrition, is a form of PEM characterized primarily by protein deficiency. This condition usually appears at the age of about 12 months when breastfeeding is discontinued, but it can develop at any time during a child's formative years.
  - It causes fluid retention (edema); dry, peeling skin; and hair discoloration.

- *Signs and symptoms:*
  - Changes in skin pigment
  - Decreased muscle mass
  - Diarrhea failure to gain weight and grow
  - Puffy eyes, moon face, fatigue
  - Hair changes (change in color or texture)
  - Increased and more severe infections due to damaged immune system
  - Irritability
  - Large belly that sticks out (protrudes)
  - Lethargy or apathy
  - Loss of muscle mass
  - Rash (dermatitis)
  - Shock (late stage)
  - Swelling (edema).

- **Marasmus:** The term Marasmus is derived from the Greek word marasmos, which means withering or wasting. Marasmus is a form of severe protein-energy malnutrition characterized by energy deficiency and emaciation.

  Primarily caused by energy deficiency, Marasmus is characterized by stunted growth and wasting of muscle and tissue.
  - Marasmus usually develops between the ages of six months and one year in children who have been weaned from breast milk or who suffer from weakening conditions like chronic diarrhea.
  - *Signs and symptoms:*
    - Severe growth retardation
    - Loss of subcutaneous fat and severe muscle wasting
    - The child looks appallingly thin and limbs appear as skin and bone shriveled body
    - Wrinkled skin
    - Bony prominence
    - Failure to thrive
    - Irritability, fretfulness and apathy
    - Frequent watery diarrhea and acid stools
    - Mostly hungry but some are anorectic
    - Dehydration

  - Temperature is subnormal
  - Edema and fatty infiltration are absent.
- **Marasmus and Kwashiorkor:** A severely malnourished child with features of both marasmus and kwashiorkor. The features of Kwashiorkor are severe edema of feet and legs and also hands, lower arms, abdomen and face. Also there is pale skin and hair, and the child is unhappy. There are also signs of marasmus, wasting of the muscles of the upper arms, shoulders and chest so that you can see the ribs.
- **Nutritional Dwarfing and Stunting:** Some children adapt to prolonged insufficiency of food-energy and protein by a marked retardation of growth. Weight and height are both reduced and in the same proportion, so they appear superficially normal.
- **Underweight Child:** Children with sub-clinical PEM can be detected by their weight for age or weight for height, which are significantly below normal. They may have reduced plasma albumin. They are at risk for respiratory and gastric infections.
- **Treatment:** Treatment strategy can be divided into three stages.
  1. **Hospital Treatment:** The following conditions should be corrected—hypothermia, hypoglycemia, infection, dehydration, electrolyte imbalance, anemia and other vitamin and mineral deficiencies.
  2. **Dietary Management:** The diet should be from locally available staple foods—inexpensive, easily digestible, evenly distributed throughout the day and increased number of feedings to increase the quantity of food.
  3. **Rehabilitation:** The concept of nutritional rehabilitation is based on practical nutritional training for mothers in which they learn by feeding their children back to health under supervision and using local foods.

Prevention

- Promotion of breastfeeding
- Development of low cost weaning
- Nutrition education and promotion of correct feeding practices
- Family planning and spacing of births
- Immunization
- Food fortification
- Early diagnosis and treatment
- Oral rehydration
- Food hygienic practices to prevent infection.

Q.2. a. Define anemia. (2)
b. Enumerate the causes of anemia. (3)
c. Explain in detail about the measures to control anemia. (10)

(A) ANEMIA

Anemia is the lack of sufficient circulating hemoglobin to deliver oxygen to tissues. Anemia has multiple causes and is often associated with other diseases. Nutritional anemia is a major problem of malnutrition affecting the most vulnerable group, e.g. pregnant and lactating women.

(B) CAUSES OF ANEMIA

- Major causes:
  - Lack of iron
  - Low quantity of folic acid
  - Low quantity of vitamin B_{12}
- Contributing causes:
  - Excessive iron loss from the body (e.g. excessive bleeding, menstruation, malaria, multiple deliveries, worm infestation, hematological disorders)
  - Protein-energy malnutrition and imbalanced diet
  - Lack of iron in diet
  - Lack of folic acid in diet
  - Excessive hemolysis and reduced formation of red blood cells
  - Use of IUD.

Signs and Symptoms of Anemia

- **Physical signs:** Headache, dizziness, tinnitus, palpitations, dyspnea on exertion, pallor of skin and mucous membrane, sore tongue, cheilosis, koilonychia
- **Behavioral signs:** Fatigue, pica (craving to eat unusual substances, e.g. sand).

(C) MEASURES TO CONTROL ANEMIA

- Correction of chronic blood loss.
- Oral or parenteral iron therapy.
  - Iron tablet 200 mg three times a day till anemia is controlled. Parenteral therapy is rarely used for those.

- Patients who cannot tolerate oral therapy, may use iron dextran or iron sorbitex.
- For preventive aspects, 180 mg of ferrous sulfate and 0.5 mg of folic acid tablets should be given everyday till the hemoglobin level reached to normal.
- Educate patient on proper nutrition and good sources of iron.
- Treatment of intestinal parasites.
- Teach patient to select balanced diet that includes green vegetables, broccoli, spinach, yeast, liver, fruits etc.
- Regular laboratory investigation.

SHORT NOTES

(5 Marks)

Q.1. Iodine deficiency disorders

Q.2. Protein-energy malnutrition

Q.3. Common nutritional deficiencies in India

Q.4. Prevention of accidents

Q.5. Cancer control measures

Q.6. Prevention of lifestyle related disease

1. IODINE DEFICIENCY DISORDERS

Iodine deficiency is a lack of the trace element iodine. It may result in goiter (so called endemic goiter), as well as cretinism, which results in developmental delays and other health problems. Iodine deficiency is an important public health issue as it is a preventable cause of intellectual disability.

Iodine is an essential trace element; the thyroid hormones thyroxine and triiodothyronine contain iodine. In areas where there is little iodine in the diet, typically remote inland areas where no marine foods are eaten, iodine deficiency is common. It is also common in mountainous regions of the world where food is grown in iodine-poor soil.

Diseases due to the deficiency of iodine have become a major nutritional problem. Some of the diseases mentioned below:

- Goiter
- Cretinism
- Myxedema.

Goiter

A goiter is a swelling of the neck or larynx resulting from enlargement of the thyroid gland (thyromegaly), associated with a thyroid gland that is not functioning properly.

Goiter which is associated with hypothyroidism or hyperthyroidism may be present with symptoms of the underlying disorder. For hyperthyroidism, the most common symptoms are associated with adrenergic stimulation: Tachycardia, palpitations, nervousness, tremor, increased blood pressure and heat intolerance.

Clinical manifestations are often related to hypermetabolism, including increased metabolism, excessive thyroid hormone, an increase in oxygen consumption, metabolic changes in protein metabolism, immunologic stimulation of diffuse goiter, and ocular changes (exophthalmos). Hypothyroid individuals may have weight gain despite poor appetite, cold intolerance, constipation and lethargy. However, these symptoms are often nonspecific and hard to diagnose.

Cretinism

Cretinism is a condition of severely stunted physical and mental growth due to untreated congenital deficiency of thyroid hormone (congenital hypothyroidism) usually due to maternal hypothyroidism. Their muscles become weak, the skin becomes thick and dry, the built becomes short and there is mental deficiency.

Myxedema

Deficiency of iodine causes lack of thyroxine, which leads to myxedema in adult. The person affected by this becomes drowsy, his hair becomes dry and rough; the skin becomes dry and yellow; voice becomes hoarse and body becomes edematous.

Preventive measures include:

- **Supplementation:** Need to start early in pregnancy. Supplement women in child bearing age.
- Iodine deficiency is treated by ingestion of iodine salts, such as found in food supplements. Mild cases may be treated by using iodized salt in daily food consumption, or drinking more milk, or eating egg yolks, and saltwater fish. For a salt and/or animal product restricted diet, sea vegetables [kelp, hijiki, dulse, nori (found in sushi)] may be incorporated regularly into a diet as a good source of iodine.

- Encourage sale of iodized salt and monitoring of its iodine content.
- Encourage community about intake of iodine and diseases caused by iodine deficiency.
- Prevention includes adding small amounts of iodine to table salt, a product known as iodized salt. Iodine compounds have also been added to other foodstuffs, such as flour, water and milk, in areas of deficiency.
- Seafood is also a well-known source of iodine.
- The recommended daily intake of iodine for adult women is 150–300 μg for maintenance of normal thyroid function; for men it is somewhat less at 150 μg.

2. PROTEIN-ENERGY MALNUTRITION

See Q.No.1 of long answer questions.

3. COMMON NUTRITIONAL DEFICIENCIES IN INDIA

While nutritional deficiencies prevail in rural areas, changes in lifestyle and the dramatic shift to unhealthy eating habits and physical inactivity has caused nutritional deficiencies to spread like an epidemic in urban areas as well. Even after sixty six years of independence, India has still to battle these top seven nutritional deficiencies.

- **Vitamin D deficiency:** Given that the best source of vitamin D is exposure to sunlight, it was believed that vitamin D deficiency is least likely to occur in people living in tropical environments like India. Surprisingly, nearly 60–80% of the Indian population is deficient in Vitamin D. Several studies have shown that vitamin D deficiency has spread across all age groups, making conditions like osteoporosis a major health problem. According to the World Health Organisation (WHO), the daily recommended allowance of Vitamin D is 600 IU/day, which you could obtain by going out in the sunlight for 15 minutes everyday.
- **Calcium deficiency:** Dietary calcium intake among Indians remains significantly low, mainly in those who have vitamin D deficiency, because its absorption is dependent on adequate levels of vitamin D. Nutritional experts note that the deficiency of a nutrient like calcium that is abundantly present in milk and milk products is a direct result of the consumption of high-calorie

foods like pizzas and burgers during early childhood years. Sticking to healthy food habits in teenage years can prevent the risk of osteoporosis and bone related disorders in adulthood.

- **Vitamin B complex deficiencies:** Although, the requirement for B vitamins is easily fulfilled with a diet rich in animal products, fruits and vegetables and cereals are milled, it is now prevalent in India. It is hard to identify B complex deficiency because neither it is killer nor does it lead to a major health problem. But, it has far-reaching effects and is carried across generations. It has increased the risk of heart disease in the past few decades, demanding more research in the field. The problem with B complex is that one micro-nutrient deficiency can lead to another. Adequate levels of vitamin B_{12} are required for conversion of inactive folate to its active form. Naturally, those without adequate levels of B_{12} are likely to suffer from folic acid deficiency.
- **Zinc deficiency:** Over the last few years, deficiency of zinc has emerged as major micronutrient deficiency. Large population is at risk, especially in the developing countries like India. It is a common in pregnant and lactating women, forming a predominant cause of death in children from rural areas.
- **Iron deficiency:** More than 75% of toddlers in India suffer from iron deficiency anemia and about 52% of young girls are severely anemic. Iron deficiency has a negative impact on brain development. It contributes greatly to maternal and child mortality. In urban areas, lack of leafy vegetables in the diet has become the primary reason for deficiency of iron resulting in anemia.
- **Iodine deficiency:** Globally, India bears the largest population of children susceptible to iodine deficiency. Although the iodine deficiency disorders (IDD) control program in India has successfully reduced the prevalence of iodine deficiency in our country, the rural population experiences iodine deficiency.
- **Vitamin A deficiency:** Vitamin A deficiency still remains a major public health nutritional problem in rural pre-school children of India. According to estimates, 250,000 to 500,000 children deficient in vitamin A become blind every year and half of them die. In India, it is more prevalent in children with vegetarian diet and often occurs along with zinc deficiency. It also makes children more susceptible to iron deficiency because of its crucial role in mobilizing iron from the site where it is stored.

4. PREVENTION OF ACCIDENTS

Accident prevention refers to the plans, preparations and actions taken to avoid or stop an accident before it happens. Accidents can be classified as unplanned and unexpected events giving increased risk of injury, ill health, death and loss of property, damage to environment or any combination of thereof. Accident prevention includes all measures taken in an effort to save lives, escape from injury, lessen the degrees of injury, reduce loss of properties, treatment and compensation costs, production and time loss, and morale loss of the concerned organization.

'Prevention is better than a cure' is an old and popular proverb, which means it is better to stop bad things from happening, than to fix them after they have already happened. Accidents are preventable, but steps must be taken to prevent them. It is a legal obligation of organizations to comply with the laws, standard practices, and safety observations to avoid emergencies and accidents.

Concepts in Accident Prevention

- **Primary prevention:** Removal of circumstances causing injury, e.g. traffic speed reduction, fitting stair gates for young children, reducing alcohol consumption.
- **Secondary prevention:** Reduces severity of injury when an accident occur, e.g. use child safety car seats, bicycle helmets, smoke alarms.
- **Tertiary prevention:** Optimal treatment and rehabilitation following injuries, e.g. effective first aid, appropriate hospital care.

Hierarchy of prevention and control measures

Risks should be avoided/eliminated and (if not possible) reduced by taking preventative measures, in order of priority. The order of priority is also known as the hierarchy of control. There different hierarchies of prevention and control measures which have been developed by different institutions. Common are five steps in the hierarchy of control in accordance to the BS OHSAS 18001 management system.

The five steps are:

- **Step 1** Elimination: Elimination of hazards refers to the total removal of the hazards and hence effectively making all the identified possible accidents and ill health impossible. The term 'elimination' means that a risk is reduced to zero without a shifting it elsewhere. Elimination is the ideal objective of any risk management. This is a permanent solution and should be attempted in the first instance.

- **Step 2** Substitution: Substitution means replacing the hazard by one that presents a lower risk. The elimination is immediately combined with a shift to another but much lower risk .
- **Step 3** Engineering Controls: Engineering controls are physical means that limit the hazard. These include structural changes to the work environment or work processes, erecting a barrier to interrupt the transmission path between the worker and the hazard. Local exhaust ventilation (LEV) to control risks from dust or fume is a common example as is separation of the hazard from operators by methods such as enclosing or guarding dangerous items of machinery/equipment. Priority should be given to measures which protect collectively over individual measures.
- **Step 4** Administrative Controls: Also known as organizational measures; it reduce or eliminate exposure to a hazard by adherence to procedures or instructions. Documentation should emphasise all the steps to be taken and the controls to be used in carrying out the activity safely.
- **Step 5** Personal Protective Equipment (PPE): PPE should be used only as a last resort, after all other control measures have been considered, or as a short-term contingency during emergency/ maintenance/repair or as an additional protective measure. The success of this control is dependent on the protective equipment being chosen correctly, as well as fitted correctly, worn at all times and maintained properly.

Prevention requires the following actions:

- Hazard identification by risk assessment
- Removal of unsafe work by research and development
- Removal of unsafe machines, tools and improvement of working conditions and environments.

Accident prevention has been traditionally based on learning from accidents and near accidents (near misses). By investigating every incident, we learn about causes and can take actions towards mitigating or removing the causes. The problem is that we have not been able to develop, in the absence of sufficiently good theories, investigation methods which would bring up all the relevant factors for prevention. An investigation may give a fairly good picture about the causes. However, this picture is usually relevant only for the specific case investigated. There may be conditions and factors which contributed to the accident whose connections the investigators do not recognize or understand. Generalizing from one accident to other situations bears a degree of risk.

The good news is that we have made considerable progress in the area of predictive safety management. A number of techniques have been developed and have become routine for industrial safety and risk analysis. These techniques allow us to study industrial production plants systematically for the identification of potential hazards and to institute appropriate action before anything happens.

5. CANCER CONTROL MEASURES

Cancer Prevention

At least one-third of all cancer cases are preventable. Prevention offers the most cost-effective long-term strategy for the control of cancer.

- **Tobacco:** Tobacco use is the single greatest avoidable risk factor for cancer mortality worldwide, causing an estimated 22% of cancer deaths per year. In 2004, 1.6 million of the 7.4 million cancer deaths were due to tobacco use.
- **Physical inactivity, dietary factors, obesity and being overweight:** Dietary modification is another important approach to cancer control. There is a link between overweight and obesity to many types of cancer such as esophagus, colorectum, breast, endometrium and kidney.
- **Alcohol use:** Alcohol use is a risk factor for many cancer types including cancer of the oral cavity, pharynx, larynx, esophagus, liver, colorectum and breast. Risk of cancer increases with the amount of alcohol consumed. The risk from heavy drinking for several cancer types (e.g. oral cavity, pharynx, larynx and esophagus) substantially increases if the person is also a heavy smoker.
- **Infections:** Infectious agents are responsible for almost 22% of cancer deaths in the developing world and 6% in industrialized countries. Viral hepatitis B and C cause cancer of the liver; human papilloma virus infection causes cervical cancer; the bacterium *Helicobacter pylori* increases the risk of stomach cancer. In some countries the parasitic infection schistosomiasis

increases the risk of bladder cancer and in other countries the liver fluke increases the risk of cholangiocarcinoma of the bile ducts. Preventive measures include vaccination and prevention of infection and infestation.

- **Environmental pollution:** Environmental pollution of air, water and soil with carcinogenic chemicals accounts for 1–4% of all cancers (IARC/WHO, 2003). Exposure to carcinogenic chemicals in the environment can occur through drinking water or pollution of indoor and ambient air.
- **Occupational carcinogens:** More than 40 agents, mixtures and exposure circumstances in the working environment are carcinogenic to humans and are classified as occupational carcinogens (Siemiatycki, et al. 2004). Those occupational carcinogens are causally related to cancer of the lung, bladder, larynx and skin, leukemia and nasopharyngeal cancer is well-documented. About 2% of leukemia cases worldwide are attributable to occupational exposures.
- **Radiation:** Ionizing radiation is carcinogenic to humans. Knowledge on radiation risk has been mainly acquired from epidemiological studies of the Japanese A-bomb survivors as well as from studies of medical and occupational radiation exposure cohorts. Ionizing radiation can induce leukemia and a number of solid tumors, with higher risks at young age at exposure.

6. PREVENTION OF LIFESTYLE RELATED DISEASE

Lifestyle diseases are diseases that are a result of the way we lead our lives on a daily basis. More work and no play, makes a lot of us prone to a host of diseases, physical ailments, and emotional problems. Some of the lifestyle related diseases are obesity, coronary heart disease, cancer, stroke, diabetes, etc.

Preventive measures include:

- Educate women, men and adolescents regarding the determinants of NCD's and various associated risk factors like unhealthy diet, physical inactivity, intake of tobacco and alcohol and stress, essentiality of iodine, etc.
- Promoting a healthy lifestyle during her regular interactions with the community.
- Assist health worker in:
  - Organizing camps/village health days on non-communicable disease themes.

- Screening of people at high risk.
- Advising patients to consult appropriate levels of health care system for diagnosis and treatment.

- Maintain a healthy diet:
  - Replace saturated and trans fats with unsaturated fats, including sources of omega-3 fatty acids. Replacing saturated fats with unsaturated fats will reduce the risk of coronary artery disease (CAD).
  - Ensure generous consumption of fruits and vegetables and adequate folic acid intake. Strong evidence indicates that high intakes of fruits and vegetables will reduce the risk of CAD and stroke.
  - Consume cereal products in their whole-grain, high-fiber form. Consuming grains in a whole-grain, high-fiber form has double benefits. First, consumption of fiber from cereal products has consistently been associated with lower risks of CAD and type 2 diabetes. Second, higher consumption of dietary fiber also appears to facilitate weight control and helps prevent constipation.
  - Limit consumption of sugar and sugar-based beverages.
  - Limit excessive caloric intake from any source.
  - Limit sodium intake. The principle justification for limiting sodium is its effect on blood pressure, a major risk factor for stroke and coronary disease.
- Increasing the availability and reducing the cost of healthy foods.
- Physical activity:
  - Develop transportation policies and a physical environment to promote walking and riding bicycles. This intervention includes constructing sidewalks and protected bicycle paths and lanes that are attractive, safe, well-lighted, and functional with regard to destinations.
  - Adopt policies that promote livable, walker-friendly communities that include parks and are centered around access to public transportation.
  - Encourage the use of public transportation and discourage overdependence on private automobiles.
  - Promote the use of stairs. Building codes can require the inclusion of accessible and attractive stairways.

SHORT ANSWER QUESTIONS

(2 Marks)

Q.1. State the classification of hypertension.

Ans. Classification of hypertension:

- **Essential hypertension:** This type of hypertension is diagnosed after a doctor notices that your blood pressure is high on three or more visits and eliminates all other causes of hypertension. Usually people with essential hypertension have no symptoms, but you may experience frequent headaches, tiredness, dizziness, or nose bleeds. Although the cause is unknown, researchers do know that obesity, smoking, alcohol, diet, and heredity all play a role in essential hypertension.
- **Secondary hypertension:** The most common cause of secondary hypertension is an abnormality in the arteries supplying blood to the kidneys. Other causes include airway obstruction during sleep, diseases and tumors of the adrenal glands, hormone abnormalities, thyroid disease, and too much salt or alcohol in the diet. Drugs can cause secondary hypertension, including over-the-counter medications such as ibuprofen (Motrin, Advil, and others) and pseudoephedrine (Afrin, Sudafed, and others).

Q.2. Mention two best sources of Iodine.

Ans. Iodine is a chemical element with symbol I and atomic number 53. Iodine and its compounds are primarily used in nutrition, and industrially in the production of acetic acid and certain polymers. Prevention includes adding small amounts of iodine to table salt, a product known as iodized salt. Iodine compounds have also been added to other foodstuffs, such as flour, water and milk, in areas of deficiency.

Its two main sources are: Sea Vegetables and Cranberries.

Q.3. Name two iodine deficiency disorders.

Ans. Iodine deficiency is a lack of the trace element iodine. It may result in goiter (so called endemic goiter), as well cretinism, which results in developmental delays and other health problems. Iodine deficiency is an important public health issue as it is a preventable cause of intellectual disability.

Iodine is an essential trace element; the thyroid hormones thyroxine and triiodothyronine contain iodine. In areas where there is little iodine in the diet, typically remote inland areas where no marine foods are eaten, iodine deficiency is common. It is also common in mountainous regions of the world where food is grown in iodine-poor soil.

Goiter: A low amount of thyroxine (one of the two thyroid hormones) in the blood, due to lack of dietary iodine to make it, gives rise to high levels of thyroid stimulating hormone (TSH), which stimulates the thyroid gland to increase many biochemical processes; the cellular growth and proliferation can result in the characteristic swelling or hyperplasia of the thyroid gland, or goiter.

Cretinism: Cretinism is a condition associated with iodine deficiency and goiter, commonly characterized by mental deficiency, deafness, squint, disorders of stance and gait, stunted growth and hypothyroidism.

Q.4. Distinguish between Kwashiorkor and Marasmus.

Ans.

Clinical features	***Marasmus***	***Kwashiorkor***
Muscle wasting	Obvious	Sometimes hidden by edema and fat
Fat wasting	Severe loss of subcutaneous fat	Fat often retained but not firmed
Edema	None	Present in lower legs, and usually in lower arms and face
Clinical features	***Marasmus***	***Kwashiorkor***
Weight for height	Very low	May be masked by edema
Mental changes	Sometimes quite and apathetic	Irritable, moaning, apathetic
Appetite	Usually good	Poor
Skin changes	Usually none	Diffuse pigmentation, sometimes flaky paint dermatitis
Hair changes	Seldom	Sparse, silky, easily pulled out
Hepatic enlargement	None	Sometimes due to accumulation of fat

Q.5. Write down the categories of mental retardation.

Ans: In intellectual disability (ID) the brain does not work properly. The brain may also not function within the normal range of both intellectual and adaptive functioning. In the past, medical professionals called this condition 'mental retardation.'

There are four levels of ID: Mild, moderate, severe, and profound. Sometimes ID may be classified as 'other' or 'unspecified.' ID involves both a low IQ and problems adjusting to everyday life. There may also be learning, speech, social, and physical disabilities.

V62.89	Borderline Intellectual Functioning	IQ 71–84
317	Mild Mental Retardation	IQ 50–55 to approximately 70
318.0	Moderate Retardation	IQ 35–40 to 50–55
318.1	Severe Mental Retardation	IQ 20–25 to 35–40
318.2	Profound Mental Retardation	IQ below 20 or 25

Q.6. What are the main causes of coronary heart diseases (CHD) in India?

Ans. Coronary heart disease (CHD) is usually caused by a build-up of fatty deposits on the walls of the arteries around the heart (coronary arteries). The fatty deposits, called atheroma, are made up of cholesterol and other waste substances. The build-up of atheroma on the walls of the coronary arteries makes the arteries narrower, restricting the flow of blood to the heart muscle. This process is called atherosclerosis. Atherosclerosis is the main cause of coronary heart disease.

Many risk factors have been associated with coronary heart disease are:

- **Hereditary:** Genetic predisposition is an important factor in the occurrence of this disease, but exact mechanism is not yet known.
- **Diabetes:** Incidence is 2–3 times more in diabetes.
- **Hypertension:** Decreased elasticity of blood vessel and tearing effect on arteries increase the incidence of this disease.
- Smoking and tobacco use increases the incidence. Both nicotine and carbon monoxide (from the smoke) put a strain on the heart by making it work faster. They also increase your risk of blood clots.
- **Diet:** Hypercholesterolemia, familial hyperlipidemia, increased levels of low density lipoproteins and increased atherogenesis.
- Obesity.

Q.7. Composition of ORS.

Ans. The reduced osmolarity ORS containing 75 mEq/L sodium, 75 mmol/L glucose (total osmolarity of 245 mOsm/L) is as effective as standard ORS in adults with cholera. However, it is associated with an increased incidence of transient, asymptomatic hyponatremia.

WHO/UNICEF ORS		ORS Osmolalities	
Ingredient	**g/L**	**Particle**	**mmol/L**
Sodium chloride	2.6	Sodium	75
Potassium chloride	1.5	Potassium	20
Glucose, anhydrous	13.5	Glucose	75
		Chloride	65
Trisodium citrate dihydrate	2.9	Citrate	10
Total	20.5	Total	245

The efficacy of ORS solution for treatment of children with acute non-cholera diarrhea is improved by reducing its sodium concentration to 75 mEq/L, its glucose concentration to 75 mmol/L, and its total osmolarity to 245 mOsm/L. The need for unscheduled supplemental IV therapy in children given this solution was reduced by 33%. In a combined analysis of this study and studies with other reduced osmolarity ORS solutions (osmolarity 210–268 mOsm/L, sodium 50–75 mEq/L) stool output was also reduced by about 20% and the incidence of vomiting by about 30%. The 245 mOsm/L solution also appeared to be as safe and at least as effective as standard ORS for use in children with cholera.

6

Demography and Population Control

LONG ANSWER QUESTIONS

Q.1. a. Define demography.

b. Discuss demographic transition.

c. Explain the scope of demography.

Q.2. a. Define population explosion.

b. Explain its effect and control measures for population explosion.

c. Role of community health nurse in control of population in India. (2 + 8 + 5 = 15 Marks)

Q.3. a. Define family planning.

b. Explain about spacing and terminal methods of family planning. (15 Marks)

SOLVED QUESTION PAPERS

Q.1. a. Define demography.
b. Discuss demographic transition.
c. Explain the scope of demography.

(A) DEMOGRAPHY

Demography is defined as the scientific study of human population which includes the study of changes in population size, its composition and distribution (Gulani KK, 2005).

Demography is the study of human population with respect to sizes, type, composition, pattern and distribution (Prabhakara GN).

It is the study of human population. It focuses its attention on three readily observable human phenomena:

1. Changes in population (growth/decline)
2. Composition of the population
3. The distribution of population in space.

It deals with five 'demographic processes', namely fertility, mortality, marriage, migration and social mobility.

(B) DEMOGRAPHIC TRANSITION

The demographic transition used to represent from high birth and death rates to low birth and death rates as a country develops from a pre-industrial to an industrialized economic system. The theory is based on an interpretation of demographic history developed in 1929 by the American demographer Warren Thompson. Thompson observed changes or transitions, in birth and death rates in industrialized societies over the previous 200 years.

The changes in the population growth rates and the effect on population can be shown on the Demographic Transition Model (Population cycle).

Stage-1 (High Fluctuating): Birth rate and death rate are both high. Population growth is slow and fluctuating. For example, typical of Britain in the 18th century and the least economically developed countries today.

Birth rate is high as a result of:

- Lack of family planning
- High infant mortality rate
- Need for workers in agriculture
- Religious beliefs
- Children as economic assets.

Death rate is high because of:

- High level of disease
- Famine
- Lack of cleanliness and sanitation
- Lack of health care
- War
- Competition for food from predators
- Lack of education

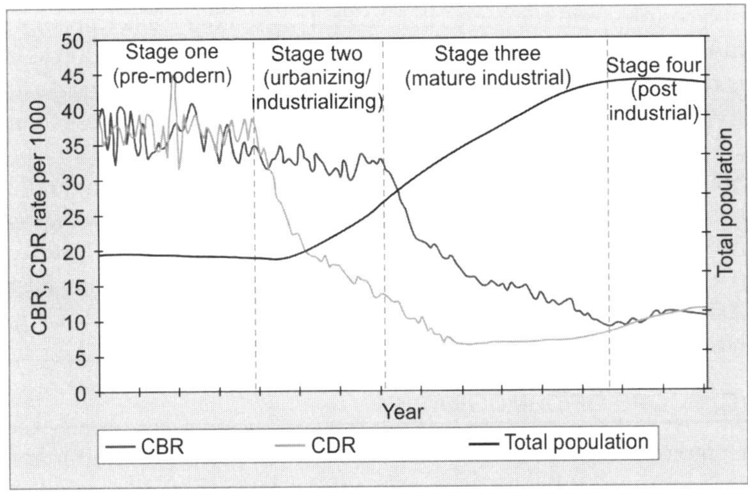

Fig. 6.1: The demographic transition model

Stage-2 (Early expanding): Birth rate remains high. Death rate is falling. Population begins to rise steadily. For example, typical of Britain in 19th century, Bangladesh, Nigeria, etc.

Reasons:

- Improved health care
- Improved hygiene
- Improved sanitation
- Improved food production and storage
- Improved transport for food.
- Decreased infant mortality rates.

Stage-3 (Late expanding): Birth rate starts to fall. Death rate continues to fall. Population rising. For example, typical of Britain in late 19th century and early 20th century, China, Brazil.

Reasons

- Family planning available
- Lower infant mortality rate
- Increased mechanization reduces need for workers
- Increased standard of living
- Changing status of women.

Stage-4 (Low Fluctuating): Birth rate and death rate both low. Population is steady. This occurs where birth rate and death rate are both low. Therefore, the total population is high and stable. Some theorist considers there are only 4 stages and that the population of a country will remain at this level. The demographic transition model is only a suggestion about the future level of a country. It is not a prediction.

Countries that are at this stage (Total fertility rate of less than 2.5 in 1997) includes United States, Canada, Brazil, etc.

Stage- 5 (Declining): The original Demographic Transition model has just four stages; however some theorists consider a 5th stage is needed to represent countries that have sub-replacement fertility (i.e. below 2.1 children per woman). Most European and many East Asian countries now have higher death rates than birth rates, e.g. Hungary, Germany are experiencing this stage.

(C) SCOPE OF DEMOGRAPHY

Demography plays a significant role in nursing. It is very important for community health nurses to know demographic aspects of community health areas.

- **Information regarding population static:** It will help nurses to plan and manage need based health care services for the community at large. The following demographic information can be collected:
  - **Total population:** This will help to determine the bulk of services and the work load which health workers are going to have.
  - **Age and sex composition:** This will help to analyze health needs, mortality and morbidity pattern, utilization of health care services and accordingly plan and manage health care services.
  - **Median age and dependency ratio:** This will help to know about the ratio of young and elderly population and adult population. This will help the nurses to determine economic determine.
  - **Socioeconomic characteristics:** These include education, marital status, occupation, income, etc. such analysis will help nurses in effective and efficient planning and management of health and nursing care at large.
  - **Family size:** Information regarding family size will help the nurses to determine socioeconomic burden on the family. Accordingly nurses will able to plan and manage family welfare services.

- **Distribution and concentration:** Distribution and concentration of population in the community will help to identify areas where services are needed most.

- **Information regarding population dynamics:** It will help the nurses to understand the changes that are taking place in the population under the influence of fertility, mortality and mitigation pattern in the community.
  - **Crude mortality rate, birth rate:** These rates will help the nurses to know natural increase in population and complete growth rate. This information will help to appreciate the need for family welfare services.
  - **Specific mortality rates:** These include age, sex, cause specific rates, case fatality and proportional mortality rates. This will help them to identify population growth at risk, specific causes of death, etc.

Q.2. a. Define population explosion.
b. Explain its effects and measures to control population explosion.
c. Role of community health nurse in control of population in India.

(A) POPULATION EXPLOSION

Population explosion refers the sudden and rapid rise in the size of population, especially human population. It is an unchecked growth of human population caused as a result of:

- Increased birth rate
- Decreased infant mortality rate
- Improved life expectancy.

Population explosion is more prominent in under-developed and developing countries than in developed countries.

(B) EFFECTS OF POPULATION EXPLOSION

The unprecedented growth of population in India during the recent year has brought about a series of serious consequences.

- **Heavy pressure on land:** Over population inevitably leads to any pressure on land. Since land is limited and fixed in supply, an increase in population can only bring more pressure on it.
- **Food shortage:** A growing population requires increasing amount of food. Even though our food production is considerably increased, it is still not possible to provide on an

average each citizen the daily required food of 18 ounce. As a result one out of every four is suffering from malnutrition and 2 out of every 4 get only half of the daily required quantum of food.

- **Housing problem:** Growing population demands housing facilities. Enough houses are not there to give shelter to the people. Every year India requires 5.9 million new houses to provide shelter to the newly addled chuck of the population. Acute shortage of houses had led to overcrowding, congestion, ill health, insanitation and often to immorality.
- **Unemployment:** In India, 12% of the people are old and 42% of them are children and have to depend on the earning of the remaining 46% of the people. Due to rapid growth of population the problem of unemployment becomes more dangerous as the years pass.
- **Illiteracy:** In India, literacy is around 36.17%. Ample number of schools and colleges are increases to meet the demand of population, even though it is not adequate. Qualities of educational standards are going down.
- **Ill health:** Indians are not only economically poor but also physically not healthy. Medical facilities that are provided are not enough to meet the growing need. Due to lack of medical facilities and nutritious food, good number of people is becoming physically and mentally handicapped. Every year along with increasing population, the number of population with ill health also increasing.
- **Environmental changes:** Due to deforestation, there is less rain, soil erosion, lack of green pastures. Exploration is going to exhaust all the underground resources within 100 years. Air pollution due to industrialization. Water pollution due to release of effluent from various factories into the water source.

Need for population control: In the world, the economic, social, cultural patterns are changing day by day.

- To maintain quality of life criteria
- To raise the standard of living
- To provide basic consumption, i.e. food, shelter, clothing, education, medical care, to control antisocial behavior
- To reduce social problem like theft, robberies
- To prevent over crowding

- To change the attitude of people towards large family size
- To overcome deep rooted religious customs, beliefs, attitudes practices favoring larger families
- To stimulate social change affecting fertility, e.g. increasing the age of marriage, women status, education, employment opportunities.

Measures suggested to control population explosion: See Q.No. 2 in the short answer questions.

(C) ROLE OF NURSE IN CONTROL OF POPULATION IN INDIA

India was the 1st country in the world to adopt a national policy on population control. Nurses have a major role to play in achieving the objectives of family planning.

- Nurses can distribute most methods of contraception and disseminate information and show films on family planning.
- They can give health talks in rural areas and while attending Mahila Mandal meetings.
- Nurses can hold family planning camps; and they can speak at parent-teacher meetings.
- In antenatal and postnatal clinics and in surgical wards, they can talk with mothers and make sure that their family planning needs are made known to the community health centers in their villages when they return.
- Nursing administrators can organize seminars, symposiums, in-service education programs and panel discussions for the nursing staff.
- Identify demographic characteristics of the adolescents and adult population and maintain data base, identify target groups and advocate the pertinent family planning methods.
- Health education to sexually active population on the STD and means to prevent them.
- Screen for sexually transmitted disease and take necessary action.
- Promote the concept of single partner among sexually active population.
- Promote the usage and distribution of condoms.
- Promote and familiarize community about contraceptive methods.

Q.3. a. Define family planning.

b. Explain about spacing and terminal methods of family planning.

(A) FAMILY PLANNING

Family planning is the planning of when to have children, and the use of birth control and other techniques to implant such plans.

Criteria for an ideal contraceptive:

- It should be safe for use means free from any kind of outside effects.
- It should be reliable.
- It should be easy to administer and convenient.
- It should be cost-effective.
- It should be culturally feasible and acceptable.

(B) SPACING AND TERMINAL METHODS OF FAMILY PLANNING

Birth control, also known as contraception and fertility control, is a method or device used to prevent pregnancy. Planning, making available, and use of birth control is called family planning. Birth control methods have been used since ancient times, but effective and safe methods only became available in the 20th century. Birth control measures are spacing and terminal method. There are mainly two birth control measures spacing and terminal methods.

Spacing Methods

It helps in prevention of pregnancy as long as they are used. These methods can help in timing and spacing of pregnancies, preventing unwanted children. These methods are temporary methods.

Natural Methods

It involves coitus interruptus, safe period and abstinence

- **Coitus Interruptus:** In this method the penis is withdrawn from the vagina before ejaculation. In this way semen is prevented from entering the uterine cavity and pregnancy does not take place. Since the penis is withdrawn and ejaculation takes place outside the vagina, this method is called coitus interruptus or withdrawal method.
- **Safe Period:** Safe period is based upon the process of ovulation and menstrual cycle which helps in determination of the safe period when coitus can be done and unsafe period when coitus can be avoided to prevent pregnancy.
- **Abstinence:** It involves complete avoidance of sexual cohabit.

Barrier Methods

Barrier methods are those methods which prevent meeting of sperms with the ovum. There are four types of barrier methods:

1. **Physical Barrier:**
   - **Condom or Nirodh:** It is a thin rubber sheath which is used by men. It is rolled over the erect penis before having sex. This rubber sheath prevents the entry of semen into the vagina. The condom must be held carefully when taking out the penis from the vagina to prevent spilling of semen into the vagina. It is available free of cost from urban or rural family welfare centers. Female condoms are also available.
   - **Diaphragm:** The diaphragm is used by women in her vagina to form a barrier in front of the cervix. The diaphragm is dome shaped and is like a shallow cap. It is made of soft synthetic rubber or plastic with a stiff but flexible rim around the edge. It is also known as Dutch Cap. Diaphragm is available in different ranging from 5–10 cm.
   - **Vaginal Sponge:** It is small polyurethane foam sponge, diffused with spermicide. The sponge is shaped in a way that it can be fitted on to the cervix and has a loop on its outer surface which can be used to pull out the sponge after use. It should be inserted before the coitus. It provides protection for 24 hours.
2. **Chemical Barrier methods:** These methods usually kill the sperms and this way chemical contraceptives help in preventing the pregnancy. The chemical contraceptives which are in use are:
   - Foam tablet aerosols
   - Cream jelly and pastes
   - Suppositories
   - Soluble films.
3. **Intrauterine Devices:** These are the devices which are placed in the uterine cavity. Earlier these devices were made up of silk worm gut, silk and gold. The three different types of IUD's generations are:
   - **First generation IUD:** These devices were made of polyethylene and are non- medicated. These are available in different sizes and shapes such as coils, spirals, loops. The lippes loop is the most popular and commonly used device. It is made of polyethylene and contains barium sulfate which makes it possible to be located when required by X-ray. The

loop is double S shaped and has an attached tail made of fine nylon threads.

- **Second generation IUD:** These are also made of polyethylene but copper is added into these. The copper enhances the contraceptive effect. Variety of copper devices are:
  - Copper-7 and copper t-200
  - Variants of T devices: TCU: 220C and TCU: 380A
  - Multi load devices: ML-CU: 250, ML-CU: 375
  - Nova T: TCU-380
- **Third Generation:** These contain hormones which are released slowly in the uterus. The hormone affects the lining of uterus and cervical mucus. It may affect the sperm. It can be of Progestasert or Levonorgestrel device.
  - **Progestasert:** It is T shaped device and contains progesterone which is a natural hormone. Progesterone is in more use than the other hormone devices.
  - **Levonorgestrel Device:** This is also a T shaped device which has levonorgestrel a synthetic steroid. It is found to be more effective. It needs to be changed after five years.

4. **Hormonal Method:** Hormonal methods of contraceptives are found to be the most effective method to prevent unwanted pregnancies. It is of two main types:
   - **Oral Pills:** There are varieties of contraceptive pills, e.g. combined pills. The pill is composed of two hormones, i.e. synthetic estrogen and progestogen in very small doses. Its action is to inhibit ovulation of ovum by blocking the secretion of gonadotropin from pituitary gland. Progestogen also thickens the mucosa of the cervix which prevents the entry of sperm into the genital canal. There are two types of pills available with the name of MALA-D, MALA-N.
     - **Progesterone only pills:** This pill is also known as mini pill. It contains only progestogen and it thickens the cervical mucus which prevents the entry of sperms into the uterine cavity. Mini pills are taken throughout the menstrual cycle and these are not used widely because of its high failure rate.
     - **Once a month pill:** It is modified combined pill. It contains long acting estrogen and short acting progestogen. These pills are not in use because experimental results

revealed high pregnancy rate and irregularity in the menstrual cycle.

- **Injectable contraceptives:** It is of two types:
    a. **Progestogen only injectable:** There are two preparations which are available; one is DMPA (Depot-medroxy progesterone acetate) and other is NET-EN.
    b. **Combined injectable contraceptives:** These contain progestogen and estrogen. The injection is given once in a month three days early or three days late.
- **Subdermal Implants:** There are two varieties. The earlier one is known as Norplant and latest one is Norplant R-2. The norplant has six small silicon rubber tubes. Each of these tubes contains 30 mg of progestogen (Levonorgestrel). The norplant R-2 has two small rods. Both of these devices are placed under the skin of the arm. The tubes or the rods allow steady diffusion of steroids into the blood stream for a period of five years to give effective contraceptive effects.
- **Vaginal Rings:** It consists of ring which contains small amount of pregestogen. The ring is fitted into the vagina for three weeks of menstruation cycle, after which it is removed for a week and then re-worn after menstruation cycle. The steroid is directly absorbed by the mucus lining of the vagina.

- **Postconceptional Methods:** These are the methods which are used after the missed period and pregnancy may or may not have occurred. This method is used in regulating and inducing the menstruation and terminating the pregnancy or aborting the fetus. It includes menstrual regulation, menstrual induction, abortion.

Terminal Methods

Sterilization is only method which gives permanent protection from conception. Either husband or wife can undergo sterilization by a simple surgical operation, i.e. vasectomy or tubectomy.

- **Vasectomy** is sterilization of male. It is very simple and minor operation which takes hardly 15–20 min. The operation involves a small cut on both sides of scrotum then a small portion of vas deferens (about 1 cm) on either side of the scrotum is cut and ligated, folded back and sutured. The operation does not affect the sexual characteristics and sex life in any form. The sperms are produces but not ejaculated along with semen.

- **Tubectomy:** It is sterilization of females. This is done by resecting a small part of fallopian tubes and ligate the tube ends. The closing of the tubes can also be done by using other methods like closing the tubes with bands, clips and electrocautery. The operation can be done through abdominal or vaginal approach. The most common abdominal procedures are laparoscopy and minilaparotomy.

Benefits of Family Planning:

- Preventing pregnancy related health risks in women.
- Reducing Infant Mortality
- Helping to prevent HIV/AIDS
- Empowering people and enhancing education
- Reducing adolescent pregnancies
- Slowing population growth.

Barriers for contraceptive use:

- **Knowledge:** Lack of sufficient education regarding the importance of reproductive health, and lack of awareness of the harmful effects of neglecting family planning on women's health and indirectly that of children.
- **Financial Attitude:** Having many children is considered a benefit as it would mean more hands to help on the field.
- **Safety net:** Due to high child mortality rate, families tend to have more children as not all survive.
- **Insurance for old age:** People have faith that children will take care of parents in their old age and so they tend to have many children.
- **Family status:** Often the social status of a family is defined by the number of children they have.
- Limited choice of methods.
- Poor quality of available resources.
- Limited access to contraception, particularly among young people, poorer segments of populations, or unmarried people.
- **Behavior:**
  - **Bias against the girl child:** In some countries like India, a girl is considered a liability as 'dowry' has to be paid to get her married. So people want to have a boy as son would be of greater use economically. Until a son is born, women keep conceiving.
  - **Rape:** Unwanted pregnancies often result from rape. According to the NCBI, It is estimated that 5% of rape victims become pregnant, that is around 32,000 a year in the US of which 32% want to keep their infants.

- **Social and public opinion:** In many societies going against public opinion leads to social ostracism. Age old traditions have formed public opinion in favor of a large family size.
- **Gender Discrimination:** In many male dominated societies, men consider it below their dignity to use contraceptive tools in their households. 'Purdah'(Veil): If the nearest available doctor is a male, women in many traditional societies in the developing world would go without medical care.
- **Religious/ethnic/racial issue:** Abortion is considered unacceptable among traditional Islamic, Christian and Hindu families.
- **Demographic barriers:** Elders are often against family planning due to age old tradition and superstition. Youngsters who want to go in for family planning risk the wrath of elders.

SHORT ANSWER QUESTIONS

Q.1. Barrier Methods of Contraception

Q.2. Measures of Population Control

Q.3. Woman Empowerment

Q.4. Population Explosion

Q.5. Small Family Norm

Q.6. Scope of Family Welfare Services

Q.7. Census

Q.8. Use of Vital Statistics

Q.9. ICDS

Q.10. Demographic Rates and Ratios

Q.11. Medical Termination of Pregnancy (MTP)

1. BARRIER METHODS OF CONTRACEPTION

Barrier methods of birth control block sperm from entering the uterus. Using a spermicide with a barrier method gives you the best possible barrier method protection.

The spermicide kills most of the sperm that enter the vagina. The barrier method then blocks any remaining sperm from passing through the cervix to fertilize an egg.

Types of barrier methods of contraception:

- **Condom:** Man's Condom is a sheath or covering, made to fit over a man's erect penis before penetration and prevents semen from coming in contact with cervix and vagina. Female Condom is a poly-urethane sheath with one flexible polyurethane ring at each end. The open ring remains outside the vagina and the symphysis like a diaphragm. It has a 0.6% breakage rate. The slippage and displacement rate is about 3% compared to 8% for male condoms.

- **Spermicides:** Foaming tablets or suppositories, melting suppositories, soluble films, jellies, and creams are used as vehicles for chemical agents that inactivate sperms in the vagina. Nonoxynol-9 is the commonest chemical agent used in these preparations.
- **Diaphragm:** This is a soft rubber cap that covers the cervix to act as a barrier. Efficacy, increases when it is used with spermicidal jelly or cream.
- **Cervical cap:** It is like the diaphragm but smaller and fits over the cervix. It is less effective in parous women.
- **Sponge:** It is a physical as well as a chemical barrier with a sustained release system for spermicide. The sponge absorbs semen and blocks the cervical canal. Commonest available preparation is 'TODAY' containing 1 gm of nonoxynol-9. It may cause allergic reaction in about 4% of users and vaginal dryness, soreness and itching in 8% of users. It does not cause toxic shock syndrome. It may enhance HIV transmission by damaging the vaginal mucosa.

Advantages of barrier methods:

- Safe, non-hormonal methods that almost every couple can use easily
- Prevent some STIs and allied conditions—pelvic inflammatory disease (PID), infertility, ectopic pregnancy and possibly cervical cancer
- Offer contraception just when needed
- Prevent pregnancy effectively if used correctly with every act of sexual intercourse
- Can be used by lactating mothers
- Can be used and discontinued without seeking a health care provider.

Disadvantages of barrier method:

- Require a high degree of motivation for regular use
- Effectiveness requires having method at hand and taking correct action before each act of sexual intercourse
- Difficult to conceal from partner

- Allergic reactions may occur in some couples with use of spermicides, latex condoms, diaphragms and caps
- Urinary tract infections are more common with the use of diaphragm and spermicides
- Accidents like slippage, breakage during coitus necessitate a `back-up' use of emergency contraception
- Careful storage is required from heat, sunlight or excessive humidity
- May embarrass some people to buy and ask partner to use these methods
- Diaphragms and cervical caps do not protect against HIV/AIDS.

2. MEASURES OF POPULATION CONTROL

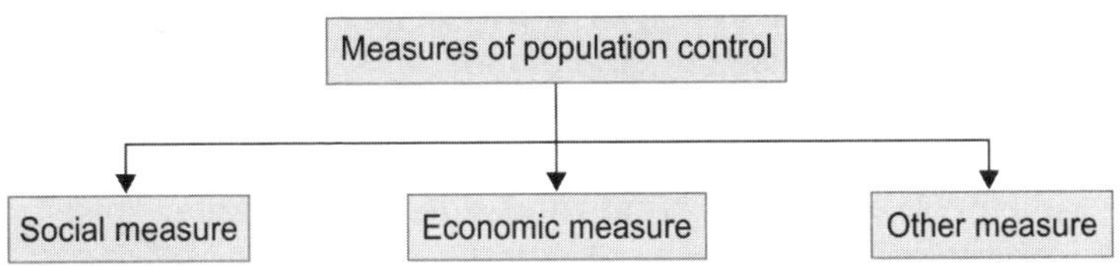

Social Measure

Population explosion is a social problem and it is deeply rooted in the society. So efforts must be done to remove the social evils in the country.

- **Minimum age of Marriage:** As fertility depends on the age of marriage. So the minimum age of marriage should be raised. In India minimum age for marriage is 21 years for men and 18 years for women have been fixed by law. This law should be firmly implemented and people should also be made aware of this through publicity.
- **Raising the Status of Women:** There is still discrimination to the women. They are confined to four walls of house. They are still confined to rearing and bearing of children. So women should be given opportunities to develop socially and economically. Free education should be given to them.
- **Spread of Education:** The spread of education changes the outlook of people. The educated men prefer to delay marriage and adopt small family norms. Educated women are health conscious and avoid frequent pregnancies and thus help in lowering birth rate.

- **Adoption:** Some parents do not have any child, despite costly medical treatment. It is advisable that they should adopt orphan children. It will be beneficial to orphan children and children couples.
- **Change in Social Outlook:** Social outlook of the people should undergo a change. Marriage should no longer be considered a social binding. Issueless women should not be looked down upon.
- **Social Security:** More and more people should be covered under-social security schemes. So that they do not depend upon others in the event of old age, sickness, unemployment, etc. with these facilities they will have no desire for more children.

Economic Measures

- **More employment opportunities:** The first and foremost measure is to raise the employment avenues in rural as well as urban areas. Generally in rural areas, there is disguised unemployment. So efforts should be made to migrate unemployed persons from rural side to urban side. This step can check the population growth.
- **Development of Agriculture and Industry:** If agriculture and industry are properly developed, large number of people will get employment. When their income is increased they would improve their standard of living and adopt small family norms.
- **Standard of Living:** Improved standard of living acts as a deterrent to large family norm. In order to maintain their higher standard of living people prefer to have a small family. According to AK Das Gupta those who earn less than ₹100 per month have on the average a reproduction rate of 3.4 children and those who earn more than ₹300 per month have a reproduction rate of 2.8 children.
- **Urbanization:** It is on record that people in urban areas have low birth rate than those living in rural areas. Urbanization should therefore be encouraged.

Other Measures

- **Late Marriage:** As far as possible, marriage should be solemnized at the age of 30 years. This will reduce the period of reproduction among the females bringing down the birth rate. The government has fixed the minimum marriage age at 21 yrs. for males and 18 yrs. for females.

- **Self-control:** According to some experts, self-control is one of the powerful methods to control the population. It is an ideal and healthy approach and people should be provided to follow. It helps in reducing birth rate.
- **Family Planning:** This method implies family by choice and not by chance. By applying preventive measures, people can regulate birth rate. This method is being used extensively; success of this method depends on the availability of cheap contraceptive devices for birth control. According to Chander Shekher, 'Hurry for the first child, Delay the second child and avoid the third.'
- **Recreational Facilities:** Birth rate will likely to fall if there are different recreational facilities like cinema theater, sports and dance, etc. are available to the people.
- **Publicity:** The communication media like TV, radio and newspaper are the good means to propagate the benefits of the planned family to the uneducated and illiterate persons especially in the rural and backward areas of country.
- **Incentives:** The government can give various types of incentives to the people to adopt birth control measures. Monetary incentives and other facilities like leave and promotion can be extended to the working class which adopts small family norms.
- **Employment to Woman:** Another method to check the population is to provide employment to women. Women should be given incentive to give services in different fields. Women are taking active part in competitive examinations. As a result their number in teaching, medical and banking, etc. is increasing rapidly. In brief by taking all these measures we can control the growth of population.

Methods for active population control

- **Contraception:** Birth control is an effective way to prevent accidental fertilization while having sex with a partner of the opposite sex. Birth control is an umbrella term for several techniques and methods use to prevent fertilization or to interrupt pregnancy at various stages.
- **Abstinence:** Sexual abstinence is the practice of refraining from some or all aspects of sexual activity for medical, psychological, legal, social or religious reasons.
- **Medical abortion:** Abortion is the termination of a pregnancy by the removal or expulsion of a fetus or embryo from the uterus,

resulting in or caused by its death. Abortion is humane and effective tool to terminate unwanted pregnancies/fetus.

- **Emigration:** Emigration is the act of leaving one's native country or region to settle in another. It is the same as immigration but from the perspective of the country of origin. Human movement before the establishment of political boundaries or within one state is termed migration.
- **Decreasing immigration:** Immigration reduction refers to a movement in the United States that advocates a reduction in the amount of immigration allowed into the country. This can include a reduction in the numbers of legal immigrants, advocating stronger action be taken to prevent illegal entry and illegal immigration, and reductions in non-immigrant temporary work visas (such as H-1B and L-1).
- **Sterilization:** It is a surgical technique leaving a male or female unable to reproduce. It is a method of birth control.
- **Euthanasia:** Refers to the practice of ending a life in a manner which relieves pain and suffering.

3. WOMAN EMPOWERMENT

Women empowerment refers to the creation of an environment for women where they can make decisions of their own for their personal benefits as well as for the society. Women Empowerment refers to increasing and improving the social, economic, political and legal strength of the women, to ensure equal-right to women, and to make them confident enough to claim their rights, such as:

- Freely live their life with a sense of self-worth, respect and dignity
- Have complete control of their life, both within and outside of their home and workplace
- To make their own choices and decisions
- Have equal rights to participate in social, religious and public activities
- Have equal social status in the society
- Have equal rights for social and economic justice
- Determine financial and economic choices
- Get equal opportunity for education
- Get equal employment opportunity without any gender bias
- Get safe and comfortable working environment

  Women have the rights to get their voices heard. While often interchangeably used, the more comprehensive concept of gender empowerment refers to people of any gender, stressing the distinction between biological sex and gender as a role. It thereby also refers to other marginalized genders in a particular political or social context.

Need to empower women:

- Under-employed and unemployed: Women population constitutes around 50% of the world population. A large number of women around the world are unemployed. The world economy suffers a lot because of the unequal opportunity for women at workplaces.
- Equally competent and intelligent: Women are equally competent. Nowadays, women are even ahead of men in many socioeconomic activities.
- Talented: Women are as talented as men. Previously, women were not allowed higher education like men and hence their talents were wasted. But nowadays, they are also allowed to go for higher studies and it encourages women to show their talents which will not only benefit her individually but to the whole world at large.
- Overall development of society: The main advantage of Women Empowerment is that there will be an overall development of the society. The money that women earn does not only help them and or their family, but it also help develop the society.
- Economic Benefits: Women Empowerment also leads to more economic benefits not to the individuals but to the society as well. Unlike earlier days when they stayed at home only and do only kitchen stuffs, nowadays, they roam outside and also earns money like the male members of the society. Women empowerment helps women to stand on their own legs, become independent and also to earn for their family which grows country's economy.
- Reduction in domestic violence: Women Empowerment leads to decrease in domestic violence. Uneducated women are at higher risk for domestic violence than educated women.
- Reduction in corruption: Women Empowerment is also advantageous in case of corruption. Women empowerment helps women to get educated and know their rights and duties and hence can stop corruption.
- Reduce Poverty: Women Empowerment also reduces poverty. Sometimes, the money earned by the male member of the family is not sufficient to meet the demands of the family. The added earnings of women helps the family to come out of poverty trap.

- National Development: Women are increasingly participating in the national development process. They are making the nation proud by their outstanding performances almost every spheres including medical science, social service, engineering, etc.

Principles of Women Empowerment: According to UN

- Establish high-level corporate leadership for gender equality
- Treat all women and men fairly at work—respect and support human rights and nondiscrimination
- Ensure the health, safety and well-being of all women and men workers
- Promote education, training and professional development for women
- Implement enterprise development, supply chain and marketing practices that empower women
- Promote equality through community initiatives and advocacy
- Measure and publicly report on progress to achieve gender equality.

Methods to empower women

- Land rights offer a key way to economically empower women, giving them the confidence they need to tackle gender inequalities. Often, women in developing nations are legally restricted from their land on the sole basis of gender.
- To allocate responsibilities to them that normally belong to men. When women have economic empowerment, it is a way for others to see them as equal members of society. Through this, they achieve more self-respect and confidence by their contributions to their communities. Simply including women as a part of a community can have sweeping positive effects.
- With the easy accessibility and affordability of e-learning (electronic learning), women can now study from the comfort of their home anywhere, anytime.
- Create safe workplaces: The workplaces should be safe for the female members of the society. People will like to send their daughters and wives to work if they are assured of safe environment at workplaces.
- Women Education: By educating women, economy of the country increases. Female education also contributes towards health and well-being of the family. Educated women are considered active in politics as well. They know their rights and are able to defend themselves better.

- Raise voice against Gender inequality: Women can be empowered by decreasing the gender inequalities or disparities in all sectors of the society especially in education sectors.
- Create more part time job opportunities for women.
- Measuring women empowerment: Women empowerment can be measured through the Gender Empowerment Measure (GEM), which shows women's participation in a given nation, both politically and economically. GEM is calculated by tracking 'the share of seats in parliament held by women'; of female legislators, senior officials and managers; and of female profession and technical workers; and the gender disparity in earned income, reflecting economic independence. It then ranks countries given this information. Other measures that take into account the importance of female participation and equality include the Gender Parity Index and the Gender-related Development Index (GDI).

4. POPULATION EXPLOSION

Population explosion refers to the rapid and dramatic rise in world population that has occurred over the last few hundred years. Between 1959 and 2000, the world's population increased from 2.5 billion to 6.1 billion people. According to United Nations projections, the world population will be between 7.9 billion and 10.9 billion by 2050.

The number of people in the world has risen from 4.4 billion people in 1980 to 6.3 billion in 2005. And it is estimated that the population could double again to nearly 11 billion in less than 40 years. This means that more people are now being added each day than at any other time in human history.

The causes of population explosion are as follows:

- **Accelerating birthrate:** Due to lack of awareness about the positive impact of using birth-control method, there has been a steady growth in birthrate.
- **Decrease in infant mortality rate:** An improvement in medical science and technology, wide usage of preventive drugs (vaccines) has reduced the infant mortality rate. There has been great improvement in medical and health care facilities during the past few decades.

- **Increase in life expectancy:** Due to improved living conditions, better hygiene and sanitation habits, better nutrition, health education, etc. The average life expectancy of human population has improved significantly.

Without these attributes present in many children's lives, they could not have survived common diseases like measles or the flu. People were able to fight and cure deadly germs that once killed them. In addition, because of the technology, people could produce more and different kinds of food. Gradually, over a period of time, these discoveries and inventions spread throughout the world, lowering death rates and improving the quality of life for most people.

Consequences: The effects of population explosion in India are as follows:

- **Over-population:** Population explosion may lead to overpopulation, i.e. a condition where population surges to a level that the earth cannot accommodate comfortably, and poses a threat to the environment.
- **Unemployment:** In developing countries like India, with a backward economy and little scope for fruitful employment, millions of people find no work to do.
- **Poverty:** High birth rate, both historically and statistically, is associated with poverty and low standard of living. It may be noted that poverty is both the cause and effect of population explosion.
- **Illiteracy:** The resources available are fixed. In theory and in practice, the total available resources are shared by the people using them. Population explosion is the key reason for illiteracy in India. People prefer engage their children in economic activities, rather than providing them education.
- **Poor Health:** If people do not get adequate food and nutrition, then they may suffer from poor health.
- **Economy:** People need food, clothes, shelter, and occupation to make their living. The demand for consumption should never exceed the production or resource limit. The economy of any country is negatively impacted, if there is massive population explosion beyond the tolerance limit.
- **Pollution and Global warming:** Too much population causes too much pressure on earth. There arises excessive demand for finished products leading to over-industrialization and over-utilization of resources.

5. SMALL FAMILY NORM

The size of the family is a matter of great importance not only for the country as a whole but also for the welfare and health of the individual, the family and the community. Our country has adopted the goal of universalizing the two-child family norm by the end of this century. The achievement of this goal has consequences both at the micro level, i.e. level of individuals and family and at the macro level, i.e. for the nation as a whole.

Need to Adopt Two-child Family Norm

Although our country has made significant progress in various developmental sectors since Independence, the fruits of these developments have not reached major segments of the poor. One important reason for this is that many of the gains have been neutralized by the rapid growth of the population. A norm in relation to family size, according to sociologists, implies a pattern which sets limits for any community's fertility behavior.

Implications of Family Size

The size of the family affects of quality of life of human beings. The quality of life does not only pertain to economic standards of living; rather it has a much wider horizon. Family size affects:

- Basic human needs
- Income and growth of the economy and savings
- Food and nutrition-quality and quantity
- Uses of land and urban public system
- Health, especially that of mother and child
- Education, particularly that of children.

Every increase in family size results in decrease in per capita food and nutrition availability and this slows down the quality of nutrition and improvement of health standards. This, in turn, has its effect on productivity of labor, which ultimately affects the overall economic development.

Advantages of a Small and Planned Family

- Reasonable gap between two children will give the mother sufficient time to replenish her body nutrients depleted due to earlier pregnancy.
- More time to participate in other fruitful activities like education, vocational training, community projects, etc.

- Can avail of better job opportunities when not tied down by small children.
- Conducive atmosphere for proper physical and psychological growth of the child.
- Planned families would gradually bring happiness, peace, harmony, prosperity.
- Improved living standards, better health, more productive labor force.
- Can provide children with better education, comfort, food, clothing, recreation, etc.
- Less chances of fetal death, birth defects, mortality during infancy and childhood.
- Small family leads to conservation of natural resources and savings.

Barriers of Small Family Norms

- Religious point: Desiring a son
- Children considered social security at old age
- Ethical uneasiness about MTP
- Lack of recreation.

Ways to Remove Barriers of Small Family Norms

- Provide recreation facilities.
- Educate poor and illiterate regarding small family norm.
- Voluntary maternity of women should have a proper place of information.
- Make Family Planning program a people's program.
- Role of voluntary organizations.

6. SCOPE OF FAMILY WELFARE SERVICES

Family welfare services are a really important part of any community health plan. WHO defines reproductive health within the framework of definition of health as 'A state of complete physical, mental and social well-being and not merely the absence of disease or infirmity, the reproductive health addresses, the reproductive processes, functions and system at all stages of life.'

This means in simpler terms that people are able to have responsible, safe and satisfying sex life with the capability to reproduce with the freedom to choose when and how to do so, if they want to. This is just the beginning of the scope of family planning. Also, nearly 4 out of 10 currently married women in

India report at least one reproductive health problem which can be a symptom of any major disease. All these together prove the urgent need for Family Welfare services in the country.

In 1951, India became the first country in the world to launch a family planning program to reduce population growth in the country. In 1997, India changed the strategy of National Family Welfare program to Reproductive and Child Health and in the ninth five-year plan (1997–2002), a total change in implementation was recommended.

Role of family welfare services are:

- To facilitate provision of antenatal and natal services to pregnant women.
- To facilitate implementation of postpartum program.
- To facilitate provision of family planning services (Basket of contraceptives, female/male sterilization, counseling, etc.)
- Implementation of UIP (Universal Immunization Program).
- Surveillance of VPD (Vaccine Preventable Diseases) Services
- Implementation of Pulse Polio Program.
- Implementation of PC and PNDT (Preconception and Prenatal Diagnostic Techniques Act, 1994, Prevention of Sex Selection) and MTP (Medical Termination of Pregnancy) Act.
- Coordination and execution of IEC activities through Mass Education Media.
- Procurement of State Specific vaccines such as MMR, Typhoid and Pentavalent Vaccines. Stocking, maintaining cold chain, disbursing vaccines and family welfare logistics to all health providing agencies in the state.
- To monitor performance and quality of family welfare activities by NGO's and release of Grant-in-Aid to them.
- To facilitate provision of Adolescent Health Services in the state of Delhi.
- Capacity building to update knowledge and skills of various categories of health functionaries by providing RCH trainings by the H&FW Training Center.

The scope of family welfare services in the country will cover the following:

- Family planning
- The dissemination of information on proper counseling and other services required by women for healthy reproduction.
- Educating population about safe delivery and postdelivery care of the mother and the baby.

- Also proper treatment of women before pregnancy.
- Health care for infants and provision of immunization against preventable diseases.
- Prevention and treatment of sexually transmitted and Reproductive Tract infections which are a leading cause of fatalities and other concerns in the country.

7. CENSUS

A census is the procedure of systematically acquiring and recording information about the members of a given population. It is a regularly occurring and official count of a particular population. The term is used mostly in connection with national population and housing censuses; other common censuses include agriculture, business, and traffic censuses. The word is of Latin origin: During the Roman Republic, the census was a list that kept track of all adult males fit for military service. The modern census is essential to international comparisons of any kind of statistics, and censuses collect data on many attributes of a population, not just how many people there are but now census takes its place within a system of surveys where it typically began as the only national demographic data collection.

A census can be contrasted with sampling in which information is obtained only from a subset of a population, typically main population estimates are updated by such intercensal estimates.

A census is often construed as the opposite of a sample as its intent is to count everyone in a population rather than a fraction.

UNFPA stated that, 'The unique advantage of the census is that it represents the entire statistical universe, down to the smallest geographical units, of a country or region. Planners need this information for all kinds of development work, including: Assessing demographic trends; analyzing socioeconomic conditions; designing evidence-based poverty-reduction strategies; monitoring and evaluating the effectiveness of policies; and tracking progress toward national and internationally agreed development goals.'

Census data offer a unique insight into small areas and small demographic groups which sample data would be unable to capture with precision.

Advantages of Census Method:

- **Higher degree of accuracy:** It provides a true measure of the population (no sampling error).
- **Intensive study:** Data collection through this method gives opportunity to the investigator to have an intensive study

about a problem. The investigator gathers a lot of information through this method.

- **Suitable for heterogeneous groups:** This method is also applicable for units for heterogeneity of difference.
- Increase confidence interval. Conducting a census often results in enough respondents to have a high degree of statistical confidence in the survey results. If you have a population of less than 1,000 individuals, you may often need to survey everyone to achieve statistical confidence.
- Maximum chance of getting negative feedback.

Disadvantages of Census Method:

- **Inconvenient:** Inconvenient in terms of time, money, etc.
- It may be difficult to enumerate all units of the population within the available time.
- It generally takes longer to collect, process, and release data than from a sample.
- Limits other possible survey opportunities. Organizations cannot ask the same people to complete a survey time and time again.

8. USE OF VITAL STATISTICS

Vital statistics are statistics on live births, deaths, fatal deaths, marriages and divorces. The most common way of collecting information on these events is through civil registration, an administrative system used by governments to record vital events which occur in their populations. Efforts to improve the quality of vital statistics will therefore be closely related to the development of civil registration systems in countries.

A vital statistics system is defined as the total process of:

- Collecting information by civil registration or enumeration on the frequency or occurrence of specified and defined vital events, as well as relevant characteristics of the events themselves and the person or persons concerned
- Compiling, processing, analyzing, evaluating, presenting, and disseminating these data in statistical form.

While the number of births and deaths can be obtained by enumeration at certain points in time (e.g. censuses and surveys), civil registration collects this information on a continuous basis and is the only source that provides individuals with a legal document.

Purposes

- **Community Health:** To describe the level of community health, to diagnose community illness and to discover solutions to health problems.
- **Administrative purpose:** It provides clues for administrative action to create administrative standards of health activities.
- **Health programmed organization:** To determine success or failure of specific health programmed or undertake overall evaluation of public health work.
- **Legislation purpose:** To promote health legislation at local, state and national level.
- **Government purpose:** To develop policies, procedure at state and central level.

Uses

- To evaluate the impact of various National Health Programs.
- To plan for better future measures of disease control.
- To explain the hereditary nature of the disease.
- To plan and evaluate economic and social development.
- It is a primary tool in research activities.
- To determine the health status of individual.
- To compare the health status of individual one nation with others.

The National Vital Statistics System

The National Vital Statistics System is one of the oldest and most successful examples of intergovernmental data sharing in public health. It is a complex system that incorporates entities at the local, state, and federal level, each with its own role. Data for vital statistics are provided through contracts between the CDC's NCHS and state- and locally-operated vital registration systems that are legally responsible for the registration of vital events: Births, deaths, marriages, divorces, and fatal deaths. The federal government's role is to compile these vital statistics and identify trends at the local, state, and national levels.

Birth Registration

Birth certificates contain a wealth of data that are important for national surveillance, research, and directing public health prevention and intervention strategies.

Death Registration

Every state is required to report all maternal deaths. Mortality statistics compiled from death certificates are used to measure health quality, set public health goals and policy, and to direct research and resources. The death certificate provides important information about the decedent, the circumstances of death, and the cause of death. In particular, maternal deaths are identified when the cause of death is coded according to the World Health Organization.

Fetal Death Reports

Completion of the fetal death report is the responsibility of the birth attendant. Importantly, several states require completion of a fetal death report for induced abortions after the fetus reaches a specific gestational age (generally 20 weeks or 24 weeks).

9. ICDS

Integrated Child Development Services (ICDS) is an Indian government welfare program which provides food, preschool education, and primary health care to children under 6 years of age and their mothers. These services are provided from Anganwadi centers established mainly in rural areas and staffed with frontline workers. In addition to fighting malnutrition and ill health, the program is also intended to combat gender inequality by providing girls the same resources as boys.

Majority of children in India have underprivileged childhoods starting from birth. The infant mortality rate of Indian children is 44 and the under-five mortality rate is 93 and 25% of newborn children are underweight among other nutritional, immunization and educational deficiencies of children in India. Figures for India are substantially worse than the country average.

ICDS was launched in 1975 in accordance to the National Policy for Children in India. Over the years it has grown into one of the largest integrated family and community welfare schemes in the world. Given its effectiveness over the last few decades, Government of India has committed towards ensuring universal availability of the program.

The predefined objectives of ICDS are:

- To raise the health and nutritional level of poor Indian children below 6 years of age.

- To create a base for proper mental, physical and social development of children in India.
- To reduce instances of mortality, malnutrition and school dropouts among Indian children.
- To coordinate activities of policy formulation and implementation among all departments of various ministries involved in the different government programs and schemes aimed at child development across India.
- To provide health and nutritional information and education to mothers of young children to enhance child rearing capabilities of mothers in the country of India.
- To provide nutritional food to the mothers of young children and also at the time of pregnancy period.

The following services are sponsored under ICDS to help achieve its objectives:

- Immunization
- Supplementary nutrition
- Health checkup
- Referral services
- Preschool non formal education
- Nutrition and Health information.

For nutritional purposes, ICDS provides 300 kilocalories (with 8–10 grams of protein) everyday to every child below 6 years of age. For adolescent girls it is up to 500 kilo calories with up to 25 grams of protein everyday.

However, World Bank has also highlighted certain key shortcomings of the program including inability to target the girl child improvements, participation of wealthier children more than the poorer children and lowest level of funding for the poorest and the most undernourished states of India.

10. DEMOGRAPHIC RATES AND RATIOS

Demographic rates and ratios help us to study the pattern of demographic changes in the population. We come to know about the trends of the population change over time. It helps in comparison of the statistics with other countries of the world. Helps to mobilize the resources and health services to the poor performing areas in relation to deaths and disease statistics

Demography is the statistical study of populations, especially human beings. As a very general science, it can analyze any kind of dynamic living population, i.e. one that changes over time or space (see population dynamics). Demography encompasses the study of the size, structure, and distribution of these populations, and spatial or temporal changes in them in response to birth, migration, ageing, and death. Based on the demographic research of the earth, earth's population up to the year 2050 and 2100 can be estimated by demographers. Demographics are quantifiable characteristics of a given population.

The Basic Measurement Tools are:

- **Rate:** Rate measures the occurrence of some particular event in a population during a given period of time. For example: Death rate:
  - *Types of rates:* The rates can be crude rates and specific rates. Crude rates are actually observed rates based on the entire population and are not reflective of any specific population group such as only females or any specific age group. For example: Crude birth rates and crude death rates.
  - *Specific Rates:* Specific rates are actual observed rates based on specific population group such as sex wise groups, age wise groups and disease wise groups or specific time periods, i.e. annual rates, monthly rates and weekly rates.
- **Ratio:** It is a measure of events which expresses a relation in size between two different factors occurring in the population and is obtained by dividing quantity of one factor with the other. It is expressed in the ratio of X:Y or X/Y, i.e. let's say here X denotes number of males and Y denotes number of females.
- **Proportion:** Proportion is a ratio which indicates the relation in magnitude of a part to the whole. The numerator is always included in the denominator. A proportion is usually expressed in percentage, e.g. number of children with scabies at certain time × 100 number of total children at same time.

Measurement Tools for Population Dynamics

- The **crude birth rate**, the annual number of live births per 1,000 people.
- The **general fertility rate**, the annual number of live births per 1,000 women of childbearing age (often taken to be from 15 to 49 years old, but sometimes from 15 to 44).
- The **age-specific fertility rates**, the annual number of live births per 1,000 women in particular age groups (usually age 15–19, 20–24, etc.)

- The **crude death rate**, the annual number of deaths per 1,000 people.
- The **infant mortality rate**, the annual number of deaths of children less than 1 year old per 1,000 live births.
- The **expectation of life** (or life expectancy), the number of years which an individual at a given age could expect to live at present mortality levels.
- The **total fertility rate**, the number of live births per woman completing her reproductive life, if her childbearing at each age reflected current age-specific fertility rates.
- The **replacement level fertility**, the average number of children women must have in order to replace the population for the next generation.
- The **gross reproduction rate**, the number of daughters who would be born to a woman completing her reproductive life at current age-specific fertility rates.
- The **net reproduction ratio** is the expected number of daughters, per newborn prospective mother, who may or may not survive to and through the ages of childbearing.

A **stable population**, one that has had constant crude birth and death rates for such a long period of time that the percentage of people in every age class remains constant, or equivalently, the population pyramid has an unchanging structure.

A **stationary population**, one that is both stable and unchanging in size (the difference between crude birth rate and crude death rate is zero).

A stable population does not necessarily remain fixed in size. It can be expanding or shrinking.

11. MEDICAL TERMINATION OF PREGNANCY (MTP)

Medical Termination of Pregnancy, 1971; (Act No. 34 of 1971)

An Act to provide for the termination of certain pregnancies by registered Medical Practitioners and for matters connected therewith or incidental thereto. Be it enacted by Parliament in the Twenty-second Year of the Republic of India as follows:

Short Title, Extent and Commencement

- This Act may be called the Medical Termination of Pregnancy Act, 1971.
- It extends to the whole of India except the State of Jammu and Kashmir.

- It shall come into force on such date as the Central Government may, by notification in the Official Gazette, appoint.

Definitions: In this Act, unless the context otherwise requires, (a) 'guardian' means a person having the care of the person of a minor or a lunatic; (b) 'lunatic' has the meaning assigned to it in section 3 of the Indian lunatic Act, 1912 (4 of 1912); (c) 'minor' means a person who, under the provisions of the Indian Majority Act, 1875 (9 of 1875), is to be deemed not to have attained his majority; (d) 'registered medical practitioner' means a medical practitioner who possesses any recognized medical qualification as defined in clause (h) of section 2 of the Indian Medical Council Act, 1956, (102 of 1956), whose name has been entered in a State Medical Register and who has such experience or training in gynecology and obstetrics as may be prescribed by rules made under this Act.

When pregnancies may be terminated by registered medical practitioners:

1. Notwithstanding anything contained in the Indian Penal Code (45 of 1860), a registered medical practitioner shall not be guilty of any offence under that Code or under any other law for the time being in force, if any pregnancy is terminated by him in accordance with the provisions of this Act.
2. Subject to the provisions of sub-section (4), a pregnancy may be terminated by a registered medical practitioner:
   a. Here the length of the pregnancy does not exceed twelve weeks if such medical practitioner is, or
   b. Where the length of the pregnancy exceeds twelve weeks but does not exceed twenty weeks, if not less than two registered medical practitioner are, of opinion, formed in good faith, that:
      i. The continuance of the pregnancy would involve a risk to the life of the pregnant woman or of grave injury to her physical or mental health; or
      ii. There is a substantial risk that if the child were born, it would suffer from such physical or mental abnormalities to be seriously handicapped.
      - Explanation 1 - Where any pregnancy is alleged by the pregnant woman to have been caused by rape, the anguish caused by such pregnancy shall be presumed to constitute a grave injury to the mental health of the pregnant woman.
      - Explanation 2 - Where any pregnancy occurs as a result of failure of any device or method used by any married woman or her husband for the purpose of limiting the

number of children, the anguish caused by such unwanted pregnancy may be resumed to constitute a grave injury to the mental health of the pregnant woman.

3. In determining whether the continuance of a pregnancy would involve such risk of injury to the health as is mentioned in sub-section (2), account may be taken of the pregnant women's actual or reasonable foreseeable environment.
4. a. No pregnancy of a woman, who has not attained the age of eighteen years, or, who, having attained the age of eighteen years, is a lunatic, shall be terminated except with the consent in writing of her guardian.
   b. Save as otherwise provided in clause (a), no pregnancy shall be terminated except with the consent of the pregnant woman.

Place where pregnancy may be terminated—no termination of pregnancy shall be made in accordance with this Act at any place other than:

a. A hospital established or maintained by Government, or
b. A place for the time being approved for the purpose of this Act by Government.

VERY SHORT ANSWER QUESTIONS

Q.1. What is Eligible Couple?

Ans. Eligible couples are those couples wherein the wife is in the reproductive age, which is generally assumed to lie between the ages of 15–45 years. There will be at least 150–180 such couples per 1000 populations in India. These couples are in need of family planning services. About 20% of eligible couples are found in the age group 15–24 years. On an average 2.5 million couples are joining the reproductive group every year. The eligible couple register is a basic document for organizing family planning work.

Q.2. Write down two objectives of Family Planning.

Ans. Family planning is the planning of when to have children and the use of birth control and other techniques to implement such plans. Other techniques commonly used include sexuality education prevention and management of sexually transmitted infection pre-conception counseling and management, and infertility management.

Family planning services are defined as 'educational, comprehensive medical or social activities which enable individuals, including minors, to determine freely the number and spacing of their children and to select the means by which this may be achieved.'

Objectives of Family Planning Program:

- Reduce infant mortality rate.
- Encourage late marriages.
- Improve women's health.
- Control of communal diseases.

Q.3. List any two actions of Copper T.

Ans: A copper IUD [ATC G02BA (WHO)] (also intrauterine device, IUD, copper-T, or coil) is a type of intrauterine device. The copper IUD is a type of long-acting reversible contraception and is one of the most effective forms of birth control.

It is on the World Health Organization's List of Essential Medicines, the most important medication needed in a basic health system.

- Copper IUDs are a form of long-acting reversible contraception and are one of the most effective forms of birth control available.
- Removal of the copper IUD should also be performed by a qualified medical practitioner. Fertility has been shown to return to previous levels quickly after removal of the device. One study found that the median amount of time from removal to planned pregnancy was three months for those women using the TCu 380Ag.

Q.4. List any four benefits of ESI Act.

Ans. 1. **Medical Benefit:** Full medical care is provided to an Insured person and his family members from the day he enters insurable employment. There is no ceiling on expenditure on the treatment of an Insured Person or his family member. Medical care is also provided to retired and permanently disabled insured persons and their spouses on payment of a token annual premium of ₹120.

2. **Sickness Benefit (SB):** Sickness Benefit in the form of cash compensation at the rate of 70% of wages is payable to insured workers during the periods of certified sickness for a maximum of 91 days in a year. In order to qualify for sickness benefit the insured worker is required to contribute for 78 days in a contribution period of 6 months.

- **Extended Sickness Benefit (ESB):** SB extendable up to two years in the case of 34 malignant and long-term diseases at an enhanced rate of 80% of wages.
- **Enhanced Sickness Benefit:** Enhanced Sickness Benefit equal to full wage is payable to insured persons undergoing sterilization for 7 days/14 days for male and female workers respectively.

3. **Maternity Benefit (MB):** Maternity Benefit for confinement/pregnancy is payable for three months, which is extendable by further one month on medical advice at the rate of full wage subject to contribution for 70 days in the preceding year.
4. **Disablement Benefit:** Temporary disablement benefit (TDB): From day one of entering insurable employment and irrespective of having paid any contribution in case of employment injury. Temporary Disablement Benefit at the rate of 90% of wage is payable so long as disability continues.
   - **Permanent disablement benefit (PDB):** The benefit is paid at the rate of 90% of wage in the form of monthly payment depending upon the extent of loss of earning capacity as certified by a Medical Board.

Q.5. Write down two advantages and disadvantages of condom usage.

Ans.

Advantages

- The condom is the best method for reducing the risk of STIs for those who choose to have intercourse. (As always, abstinence is the only 100% guarantee.)
- Allows men to share responsibility for pregnancy prevention and protection against STDs.
- Can be easily obtained and does not require a prescription.

Disadvantages

- Some people are allergic to latex. Polyurethane condoms can be used as an alternative.
- Some individuals argue that condoms reduce sensitivity and pleasure during intercourse.
- Some people dislike interrupting sex to put it on.
- Condoms may break if they are put on incorrectly.

Q.6. What are Intrauterine Devices?

Ans. An intrauterine device (IUD or coil) is a small contraceptive device, often 'T'-shaped, often containing either copper or levonorgestrel, which is inserted into the uterus. They are one form of long-acting reversible contraception which are the most effective types of reversible birth control. Failure rates with the copper IUD is about 0.8% while the levonorgestrel IUD has a failure rate of 0.2% in the first year of use.

Copper IUDs primarily work by disrupting sperm mobility and damaging sperm so that they are prevented from joining with an egg. Copper acts as a spermicide within the uterus, increasing levels of copper ions, prostaglandins, and white blood cells within the uterine and tubal fluids. The increased copper ions in the cervical mucus inhibit the sperm's motility and viability, preventing sperm from travelling through the cervical mucus, or destroying it as it passes through. Copper can also alter the endometrial lining, but studies show that this alteration can prevent implantation, but not disrupt implantation.

Q7. Define Population Pyramid?

Ans. Population pyramid is a graphical illustration that shows the distribution of various age groups in a population which normally forms the shape of a pyramid.

Types of population pyramid:

- Stationary pyramid: A population pyramid showing an unchanging pattern of fertility and mortality
- Constructive pyramid: A population pyramid showing lower percentage of younger people.
- Expansive pyramid: In this, there is a broad base indicating a high proportion of children. Growth of population is increasing.

Q8. Census of India?

Ans: The decennial Census of India has been conducted 15 times, as of 2011. It has been conducted every 10 years, beginning in 1872. Post 1949, it has been conducted by the Registrar General and Census Commissioner of India.

Key Facts of Census of India (2011)

- 35 states and UTs; 640 districts; 6.41 lacs villages
- Total Population: 1210.1 million
- Sex ratio: 940

- India is 2nd rank in population with 17.64% decadal growth and China is 1st rank with decadal growth 19% (over 1.35 billion).
- Most populous state: Uttar Pradesh (199,812,341)
- Least populous state: Sikkim (610,577)
- Rate of growth of population of India: 17.64%
- State having highest fertility rate: Meghalaya
- Literacy rate in India: 74.04%

Q9. Define Growth Rate?

Ans: Growth rate is defined as the change in population overtime, and can be quantified as the change in the number of individuals in a population per unit time.

Growth rate can be decadal or annual growth rate

- Decadal growth rate: Change in population over a decade
- Annual growth rate: Crude birth rate minus crude death rate.

Q.10. Who conducted census of India? When was the last census undertaken in India?

Ans. Registrar General and Census Commissioner, Ministry of Home affairs, Government of India conduct census of India. Last census was undertaken in 2011.

Papers → Practice what you need to study → Original question papers

Rajiv Gandhi University of Health Sciences, Karnataka

Second Year BSc Nursing Degree Examination—Feb/March 2011

Time: Three Hours **Max. Marks: 75**

Community Health Nursing I (RS 2 and RS 3)
QP CODE: 1764

Your answers should be specific to the questions asked
Draw neat labeled diagrams wherever necessary

Long Essays (Answer any Two) 2 × 10 = 20 Marks

Q.1. Describe the determinants of health.
Q.2. Discuss the different levels of prevention.
Q.3. (a) Explain the epidemiology of poliomyelitis.
(b) Discuss the control and preventive measures of polio.
(c) Measures for polio eradication.

Short Essays (Answer any Seven) 7 × 5 = 35 Marks

Q.4. Explain the rapid sand filtration method
Q.5. Cold chain
Q.6. Epidemiological triad
Q.7. Oral rehydration therapy
Q.8. Protein energy malnutrition
Q.9. Intrauterine devices
Q.10. Population explosion
Q.11. Sanitary well
Q.12. Influenza

Short Answers 10 × 2 = 20 Marks

Q.13. Quarantine
Q.14. Promotion of health
Q.15. Couple protection rate
Q.16. Safe period
Q.17. Pasteurization
Q.18. Vitamin 'A' prophylaxis
Q.19. Monteux test
Q.20. Chemoprophylaxis
Q.21. Herd immunity
Q.22. Obesity

Rajiv Gandhi University of Health Sciences, Karnataka

Second Year BSc Nursing Degree Examination—Feb 2010

Time: Three Hours **Max. Marks: 75**

Community Health Nursing I (RS 2)
QP CODE: 1764

Your answers should be specific to the questions asked
Draw neat labeled diagrams wherever necessary

Long Essays (Answer any Two) **2 × 10 = 20 Marks**

Q.1. (a) Define community health
(b) Describe the concepts and dimensions of health
Q.2. Discuss the family welfare programme in India and explain the role of nurse in family welfare programme
Q.3. Define the epidemiology and explain nursing management of dengue and briefly discuss the control measures

Short Essays (Answer any Seven) **7 × 5 = 35 Marks**

Q.4. Women empowerment
Q.5. Functions of family
Q.6. Epidemiological triad
Q.7. Marriage system in India
Q.8. Family budgeting
Q.9. Determinants of health
Q.10. Protein energy malnutrition
Q.11. Prevention of food poisoning
Q.12. Control of viral hepatitis

Short Answers **10 × 2 = 20 Marks**

Q.13. Define stroke
Q.14. Demography
Q.15. Tetanus vaccine
Q.16. Tubectomy
Q.17. Target free approach
Q.18. Disadvantages of nuclear family
Q.19. Infant mortality rate
Q.20. Zoonoses
Q.21. IUCD
Q.22. Mental health

Rajiv Gandhi University of Health Sciences, Karnataka

Second Year BSc Nursing Degree Examination—Aug/Sept 2009

Time: Three Hours **Max. Marks: 75 Marks**

Community Health Nursing I (RS 2)
QP CODE: 1764

Your answers should be specific to the questions asked
Draw neat labeled diagrams wherever necessary

Long Essays (Answer any Two) **2 × 10 = 20 Marks**

Q.1. (a) Define demography
(b) Explain the methods of collection, analysis and interpretation of demographic data

Q.2. (a) Define epidemiology
(b) Explain disease transmission

Q.3. Describe the determinants of health

Short Essays (Answer any Seven) **7 × 5 = 35 Marks**

Q.4. Anemia
Q.5. Sociocultural aspects of community
Q.6. Levels of prevention
Q.7. Importance of exercise and rest
Q.8. Safe period
Q.9. Prevention of food adulteration
Q.10. Promotion of small family norm
Q.11. Dimensions of health
Q.12. Prevention and control of AIDS

Short Answers **10 × 2 = 20 Marks**

Q.13. Rabies
Q.14. Oral contraceptives
Q.15. Juvenile diabetes
Q.16. Trachoma
Q.17. Vasectomy
Q.18. Active immunity
Q.19. Census
Q.20. Hygiene
Q.21. Crude birth rate
Q.22. Eligible couple

Rajiv Gandhi University of Health Sciences, Karnataka

Second Year BSc Nursing Degree Examination—March/April 2008

Time: Three Hours **Max. Marks: 80**

Community Health Nursing I (RS)
QP CODE: 1686

Your answers should be specific to the questions asked
Draw neat labeled diagrams wherever necessary

Long Essays (Answer any Two) 2 × 10 = 20 Marks

Q.1. State how to identify a family with health risk factors and what nursing intervention provided at primary, secondary and tertiary level of care.
Q.2. Discuss the health aspects of family planning; explain the role of community health nurse in family welfare service.
Q.3. Discuss the factors influencing hygienic practices and write principles relevant to personal hygiene.

Short Essays (Answer any Eight) 8 × 5 = 40 Marks

Q.4. Principles of home visiting
Q.5. Importance of sex education
Q.6. Health survey
Q.7. Mental health
Q.8. Purposes of using records and reports
Q.9. Principles used in bag technique
Q.10. APGAR score
Q.11. Methods of fertility
Q.12. Causes of maternal mortality in India
Q.13. Family functions

Short Answers 10 × 2 = 20 Marks

Q.14. Define community diagnosis
Q.15. Small for date-babies
Q.16. AIDS prevention
Q.17. Principles of working in community
Q.18. Baby friendly hospitals

Q.19. Symbol of under five clinic
Q.20. Growth monitoring
Q.21. Child survival index
Q.22. Importance of physical exercises
Q.23. Define nursing care plan

Post Graduate Institute of Medical Sciences College of Nursing, Rohtak, Haryana

BSc Nursing IInd Year Supplementary, 2016

March, 2016/1524

Time: Three Hours **Max. Marks: 75**

Community Health Nursing I

Note: Attempt all questions. Attempt all parts of a question at one place.

Q.1 (a) Explain analytical epidemiology in detail **10 + 5 = 15**
(b) Write down the formulae of
(i) Perinatal mortality rate
(ii) Neonatal mortality rate

Q.2 (a) Describe the mechanism of disposal of dead bodies in India **5 + 10 = 15**
(b) Explain the role of security and purchasing power in financial management

Q.3 (a) Write down the epidemiology of severe acute respiratory syndrome (SARS) and write the nursing management of SARS **10 + 5 = 15**
(b) Write the epidemiology of leptospirosis

Q.4 (a) Write the epidemiology and nursing management of mental illness **10 + 5 = 15**
(b) What is the scope of demography?

Q.5 Write short notes on any three of the following: **5 × 3 = 15**
(a) Women empowerment
(b) Emergency contraception
(c) Infrastructural facilities and linkages
(d) Promotion of health
(e) Scope of epidemiology
(f) Status of children and society

Post Graduate Institute of Medical Sciences College of Nursing, Rohtak, Haryana

BSc Nursing IInd Year Annual, 2015

August, 2015/1524

Time: Three Hours **Max. Marks: 75**

Community Health Nursing I

Note: Attempt all questions. Attempt all parts of a question at one place.

Q.1 (a) Enlist the aims of epidemiology **5 + 10 = 15**
(b) Describe descriptive epidemiology in detail

Q.2 (a) What is eugenics? **5 + 10 = 15**
(b) Describe all the acts regulating the environment

Q.3 (a) Write the epidemiology of diarrheal disease and explain the nursing management of diarrheal diseases. **10 + 5 = 15**
(b) What is the status of elderly people in India?

Q.4 (a) Write the epidemiology of stroke and explain the nursing management of a stroke patient **10 + 5 = 15**
(b) Describe the scope of demography

Q.5 Write short notes on any three of the following: **5 × 3 = 15**
(a) Chemical methods of contraception
(b) Population explosion
(c) Concept of epidemiology
(d) Noise pollution
(e) Sewage disposal
(f) Food preservation

Post Graduate Institute of Medical Sciences College of Nursing, Rohtak, Haryana

BSc Nursing IInd Year Annual

August, 2014/1524

Time: Three Hours **Max. Marks: 75**

Community Health Nursing I

Note: Attempt all questions. Attempt all parts of a question at one place.

Q.1 (a) Define community **2 + 4 + 7 = 13**
(b) Write about the physical environment responsible for sound health
(c) Explain about maintenance of food hygiene

Q.2 (a) Discuss 'hygiene' **2 + 10 = 12**
(b) Discuss about physical activity responsible for maintenance of positive health

Q.3 (a) Define 'epidemiology' **2 + 10 = 12**
(b) Discuss about levels of prevention of disease

Q.4 (a) Define population explosion **3 +10 = 13**
(b) Discuss its impact on social and economic development of individual and society

Q.5 Write short notes on any five of the following: **5 × 5 = 25**
(a) Demography
(b) First aid for sun-stroke
(c) Zoonosis
(d) Iodine deficiency
(e) Mental illness
(f) Prevention of malaria
(g) Morbidity and mortality
(h) Dynamics of disease
(i) Acts regulating food hygiene

Post Graduate Institute of Medical Sciences College of Nursing, Rohtak, Haryana

BSc Nursing IInd Year Annual July, 2013/1524

Time: Three Hours **Max. Marks: 75**

Community Health Nursing I

Note: Attempt all questions. Attempt all parts of a question at one place.

Q.1 (a) Define community health nursing **2 + 6 + 7 = 15**
(b) Discuss the determinants of health
(c) Explain your role as a nurse in promotion of health in the community

Q.2 (a) Define epidemiology **2 + 7 + 6 = 15**
(b) Discuss the level of prevention of disease with suitable examples
(c) Describe epidemiological triad with example

Q.3 (a) Define air pollution **2 + 7 + 6 = 15**
(b) Enlist the health hazards due to air pollution
(c) Describe the role of a nurse in prevention of airborne diseases

Q.4 (a) Explain the concept of demographic cycle **7 + 8 = 15**
(b) Discuss the methods of family planning that can be advised to group of people

Q.5 Write short notes on any three of the following: **5 × 3 = 15**
(a) Prevention of diabetes
(b) Food hygiene
(c) Women empowerment
(d) Noise pollution
(e) Dengue fever

Post Graduate Institute of Medical Sciences College of Nursing, Rohtak, Haryana

BSc Nursing IInd Year Annual
July, 2012/1524

Time: Three Hours **Max. Marks: 75 Marks**

Community Health Nursing I

Note: Attempt all questions.

Q.1 Define health. Describe dimensions of health. Explain the factors influencing health. **2 + 5 + 8 = 15**

Q.2 (a) Explain the concept of safe and wholesome water **4 + 6 + 5 = 15**

(b) Identify the sources of water pollution and enlist the water-borne disease.

(c) Discuss the role of a nurse in prevention of water borne disease

Q.3 (a) Define demography. Discuss demographic stages **5 + 10 = 15**

(b) Explain the impact of population growth on the community

Q.4 (a) Explain the meaning of epidemiology **5 + 10 = 15**

(b) Briefly discuss the epidemiological factors of cardiovascular diseases and role of nurse in controlling cardiovascular diseases in the community

Q.5 Write short notes on any three of the following: **5 × 3 = 15**

(a) Epidemiological measurements
(b) Air pollution
(c) Food hygiene
(d) MTP Act
(e) Obesity
(f) Noise

Baba Farid University of Health Sciences Faridkot, Punjab

Second Year BSc Nursing Degree Examination BF/2014/01

Time: Three Hours **Max. Marks: 75**

Community Health Nursing I
New Scheme wef 2006

Note: Attempt all questions

Q.1. (i) (a) Define community health nursing. [3]
(b) Explain the concepts of community health nursing. [5]
(c) Discuss the dimensions of health. [7]

OR

(ii) (a) What is typhoid fever? [3]
(b) List down the signs and symptoms of typhoid fever. [4]
(c) Describe the preventive measures for a patient with typhoid. [8]

Q.2. (a) Describe the determinants of health. [2]
(b) Explain any two acts regulating food hygiene. [6]
(c) What is the role of National Pollution Control Board in regulating environment? [7]

Q.3. (a) Explain epidemiological triad in detail. [5]
(b) How will you calculate morbidity and mortality rates in community? [5]

Q.4. (a) What is diphtheria? [2]
(b) List down the signs and symptoms and home management of diphtheria. [8]

Q.5. Write short notes on any *five* of the following : [5 × 5 = 25]
(a) AIDS.
(b) Hypertension.
(c) Obesity.
(d) Community survey.
(e) Ventilation.
(f) Women empowerment.
(g) Hygiene.

Baba Farid University of Health Sciences Faridkot, Punjab

Second Year BSc Nursing Degree Examination-BF/2013/07

Time: Three Hours **Max. Marks: 75**

Community Health Nursing I
New Scheme wef 2006

Note: Attempt all questions

Q.1.(a) Define demography. [3]
(b) Methods of data collection. [5]
(c) What all points you will remember while assessing the survey reports? [7]

OR

Q.2.(a) What is pneumonia? [3]
(b) List down the signs and symptoms of pneumonia. [4]
(c) Describe the preventive measures for a child in community area. [8]

Q.3.(a) Define population control. [2]
(b) Describe the methods of population control. [6]
(c) How will you promote small family in community area. [7]

Q.4. If you are posted in community for assessment of environmental pollution.
(a) How will you control arthropods and rodents. [5]
(b) Health education on disposal of waste from houses. [5]

Q.5.(a) What do you understand by diarrheal disease? [3]
(b) Discuss the role of nurse in prevention of diarrheal disease. [7]

Q.6.Write short notes on any five of the following: [5 × 5 = 25]
(a) Malaria.
(b) Leprosy.
(c) Poliomyelitis.
(d) Concepts of community health nursing.
(e) Rheumatic heart disease.
(f) Role of nurse in meningitis.
(g) Epidemic investigation.

Baba Farid University of Health Sciences Faridkot, Punjab

Second Year BSc Nursing Degree Examination-BF/2012/08

Time: Three Hours **Max. Marks: 75**

Community Health Nursing I
New Scheme wef 2006

Note: Attempt all questions

Q.1. (a) Define epidemiology. [2]
(b) Write down the scope of epidemiological study. [4]
(c) Discuss in brief about descriptive epidemiology as a method of survey. [9]

OR

Q.1. (a) Explain health as a dynamic phenomenon. [3]
(b) Discuss how knowledge of health dimension is required by a nurse in identifying health needs of an individual. [6]
(c) Discuss in brief about determinants of health. [6]

Q.2 You are working as a community health nurse in a health agency. You have detected few cases of suspected tuberculosis during your home visit.
(a) How would you diagnose a case of tuberculosis? [3]
(b) What is the current treatment of tuberculosis? [5]
(c) Write your function as a community health nurse in prevention and control of tuberculosis. [7]

Q.3. (a) Define hypertension. [1]
(b) What are the risk factors of hypertension? [4]
(c) Briefly describe the primary and secondary level of prevention of hypertension. [5]

Q.4. (a) Name the six arthropod borne diseases of public health importance.
(b) Explain briefly the various methods of mosquito control with reference to National Malaria Control of India.
[3 + 7 = 10]

Q.5. Write short notes on any *five* of the following: **[5 × 5 = 25]**
(a) Levels of prevention.
(b) Food hygiene.

(c) Road to health growth chart.
(d) Sources of demographic data.
(e) Barrier methods of family planning.
(f) Characteristics of a mentally healthy person.
(g) Sources of air pollution.

Baba Farid University of Health Sciences, Faridkot, Punjab

Second year BSc Nursing Degree Examination-BF/2011/07

Time: Three Hours **Max. Marks: 75**

Community Health Nursing I
New Scheme wef 2006

Note: Attempt all questions

Q.1. (a) Define health. [2]
(b) List the various dimensions of health. [3]
(c) Describe any *three* dimensions of health in detail with suitable examples. [10]

OR

Q.1. (a) Define community health nursing. [2]
(b) What do you understand by 'positive health'? [3]
(c) Explain the various levels of disease prevention with appropriate examples. [10]

Q.2. (a) Write the factors that have led to increased population in India. [7½]
(b) Describe what steps have been taken by the Government of India for population control. [7½]

Q.3. (a) What is the epidemiology of hepatitis 'A'? [3]
(b) Prepare a health-talk plan for the prevention of hepatitis 'A' in the community. [7]

Q.4. (a) List the causes of malnutrition in preschool children. [3]
(b) Describe the role of a community health nurse in prevention of malnutrition in children. [7]

Q.5. Write short notes on any *five* of the following: [5 × 5 = 25]
(a) Control of blindness.
(b) Healthful housing.
(c) Food adulteration.
(d) Descriptive epidemiology.
(e) DOTS therapy.
(f) Fly control measures.
(g) Sources and biological hazards of radiation.

Baba Farid University of Health Sciences Faridkot, Punjab

Second Year BSc Nursing Degree Examination-BF/2010/12

Time: Three Hours **Max. Marks: 75 Marks**

Community Health Nursing I
New Scheme wef 2006

Note: Attempt all questions

Q.1. a. Define `small-family-norm'.
b. Discuss the role of a community health nurse for population control. **[3 + 8 = 11]**

Q.2. a. Define 'epidemiology'.
b. Write about role of a community health nurse towards control and prevention of cholera in community. **[3 + 8 = 11]**

Q.3. a. List the different types of anemia.
b. Discuss the role of community health nurse towards prevention of iron deficiencey anemia in community. **[4 + 8 = 12]**

Q.4. a. List the signs and symptoms of disease tuberculosis.
b. Prepare a health-talk plan for prevention of tuberculosis in community. **[3 + 8 = 11]**

Q.5. Write short notes on any *three* of the following:
a. Prevention of hookworm infection.
b. Dynamics of disease.
c. Ventilation.
d. Immunization.
e. Sanitation.
f. Methods of data collection and interpretation. **[10 × 3 = 30]**

Baba Farid University of Health Sciences
Faridkot, Punjab

Second Year BSc Nursing Degree
Examination-BF/2009/11

Time: Three Hours **Max. Marks: 75 Marks**

Community Health Nursing I
New Scheme wef 2006

Note: Attempt all questions

Q.1. a. What are the agent, host and environmental factors in causation of filaria? [7]
b. Discuss the measures to prevent and control of filaria in urban slum community. [8]

Q.2. a. List the criteria of safe and wholesome water.
b. Write health hazards due to contaminated water.
c. Explain purification of water on a small scale.
[2 + 4 + 9 = 15]

Q.3. Explain any *two* of the following:
a. Causes of population explosion in India.
b. Disposal of dead bodies after earthquake.
c. Promotion of health. [$7^1/_2$ × 2 = 15]

Q.4. a. List the common sexually transmitted diseases. [2]
b. Explain the host factors of HIV infection. [6]
c. Describe the measures to prevent and control HIV/AIDS infection. [7]

Q.5. Write short notes on any *three* of the following:
a. Fluorosis.
b. Importance of recreation and sleep in life.
c. National pollution control board.
d. Drugs and cosmetic Act.
e. Immunity. [5 × 3 = 15]

Baba Farid University of Health Sciences Faridkot, Punjab

Second Year BSc Nursing Degree Examination-BF/2009/06

Time: Three Hours **Max. Marks: 70 Marks**

Community Health Nursing I
(Old Scheme)

Note: Attempt all questions

Q.1. (a) Explain milestones in the history of community health in India. [7]
(b) Discuss principles of community work. [7]
Q.2. (a) Explain epidemiological triad in causation of diseases. [6]
(b) Describe levels of prevention with example. [8]
Q.3. (a) Explain advantages of record keeping and reporting of vital statistics.
(b) Describe vital events that affect health services. [7]
Q.4. (a) Discuss nursing profession—a sociological interpretation. [6]
(b) Explain role of traditional health functionaries in community health. [8]
Q.5. (a) Explain objective and scope of family welfare programme. [9]
(b) Comment on demographic indicators in India. [5]
Q.6. Write short note on any *two:* [7 + 7 = 14]
a. Effects of poor housing
b. Health legislation
c. Prevention of home accidents
d. Milk hygiene
e. Nature of culture

Kerala University, Kerala

Second Year BSc Nursing Degree Examination

(Model Question Paper)

Time: Three Hours **Max. Marks: 75**

Community Health Nursing

Essays [20]

Q.1. Describe the spectrum of health. Explain the determinants of health. [3 + 7 = 10]

Q.2. Define epidemiology. Describe the epidemiology of tuberculosis and its preventive measures. [1 + 4 + 5 =10]

Short Notes [7 × 5 = 35]

Q.3. Pasteurization of milk

Q.4. Modern sewage treatment

Q.5. Role of community health nurse in IEC

Q.6. Elements of primary health care

Q.7. Population explosion

Q.8. Food hygiene

Q.9. Advantages of home visit

Define the Following: [5 × 2 = 10]

Q.10. Community health nursing

Q.11. Demography

Q.12. Health education

Q.13. Malnutrition

Q.14. Eligible couple

Differentiate Between the Following: [5 × 2 = 10]

Q.15. Infective hepatitis—serum hepatitis

Q.16. Smallpox—chickenpox

Q.17. Tubectomy—vasectomy

Q.18. Hospital nursing—community health nursing

Q.19. Shallow well—deep well

Annexures

ANNEXURE

1

Census of India 2011

1. Census 2011 was released in New Delhi on 31st March 2011 by Union Home Secretary GK Pillai and RGI C Chandramouli.
2. Census 2011 was the 15th census of India and 7th census after Independence.
3. The motto of census 2011 was 'Our Census, Our Future'.
4. Total estimated cost of the census was INR2200 crore (US$350 million).
5. First census in 1872.
6. Total population—1,210,854,977 (1.21 billion).
7. India in 2nd rank in population with 17.64%. Decadal growth and China is 1st rank with decadal growth 19% (over 1.35 billion).
8. World population is 7 billion.
9. Increase in population during 2001–2011 is 181 million.
10. Most populous state: Uttar Pradesh (199,812,341).
11. Least populous state: Sikkim (610,577).
12. Sex ratio: 940 females per 1000 males.
13. Growth rate: Decadal growth rate: 17.64% and annual growth rate is 1.64%.

ANNEXURE 2

Demography and Fertility Indicators

S.no.	Demographic and fertility indicators	Level
1	Crude birth rate (CBR)	21 per 1000 midyear population (SRS 2014)
2	Crude death rate (CDR)	6.7 per 1000 midyear population (SRS 2014)
3	Infant mortality rate (IMR)	39 per 1000 live births (SRS 2014)
4	Under 5 mortality rate (U5MR)	45 per 1000 live births (SRS 2014)
5	Sex ratio at birth	906 in 2012–2014 (SRS 2014)
6	Total fertility rate (TFR)	2.3 (SRS 2014)
7	General fertility rate (GFR)	77.6 (SRS 2014)
8	Gross reproduction rate (GRR)	77.6 (SRS 2014)
9	Maternal mortality rate (MMR)	178 per 100,000 live births (SRS 2012)
10	Female sterilization	3951972 (annual report MOHFW 2015–16)
11	Male sterilization	78362 (annual report MOHFW 2015–16)
12	IUCD	5277460 (annual report MOHFW 2015–16)

ANNEXURE **3**

Total Population and Decadal Growth Rates of India

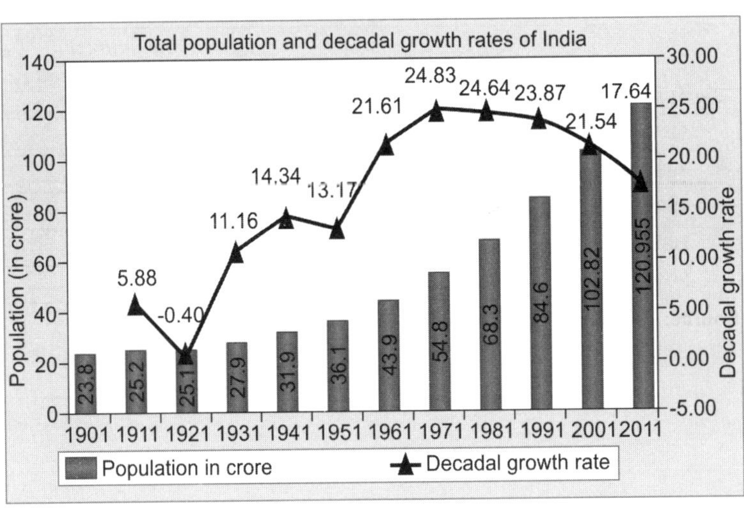

Source: Annual Report MOHFW 2015–16

ANNEXURE 4

Growth of Population in India

Census year	Population (in crores)	Decadal growth (%)	Average annual exponential growth (%)
1971	54.82	24.80	2.20
1981	68.33	24.66	2.22
1991	84.64	23.87	2.16
2001	102.87	21.54	1.97
2011	121.02	17.64	1.64

Source: Annual Report MOHFW 2015–16

ANNEXURE 5

Achievements of Health and Family Program

S. no.	*Parameter*	*1951*	*1981*	*1991*	*2001*	*2013 (latest available)*
1	Crude birth rate (per 1000 population)	40.8	33.9	29.5	25.4	21.4
2	Crude death rate (per 1000 population)	25.1	12.5	9.8	8.4	7.0
3	Total fertility rate (per women)	6.0	4.5	3.6	3.1	2.3 (2013)
4	Maternal mortality ratio (per 1000 live births)	NA	NA	437 (1992–93) NFHS	301 (2001–3) SRS	167 (2011–13) SRS
5	Infant mortality rate (per 1000 live births)	146 (1951–61)	110	80	66	40
6	Expectation of life at birth	–	55.4 (1981–85) Mid-year 1983	59.4 (1989–93) Mid-year 1991	63.4 (1999–3) Mid-year 2001	67.5 (2009–13) Mid-year 2011

Source: Office of Registrar General and Census Commissioner, India, Ministry of Home Affairs.

ANNEXURE 6

Kuppuswami Scale for Socio-economic Status (Urban Families)

(A)	Education	Score
1	Profession or honors	7
2	Graduate or postgraduate	6
3	Intermediate or post high school diploma	5
4	High school certificate	4
5	Middle school certificate	3
6	Primary school certificate	2
7	Illiterate	1
(B)	***Occupation***	***Score***
1	Professional	10
2	Semi professional	6
3	Clerical, shop owner, farmer	5
4	Skilled worker	4
5	Semi skilled worker	3
6	Unskilled worker	2
7	Unemployed	1
(C)	***Family income per month (₹)****	***Score***
1	≥ 31,507	12
2	15,754–31,506	10
3	11,817–15,753	6
4	7,878–11,816	4
5	4,727–7,877	3

6	1,590–4,726	2
7	≤ 1,589	1
(D)	***Socio-economic class***	***Score***
1	Upper	26–29
2	Upper middle	16–25
3	Lower middle	11–15
4	Upper lower	05–10
5	Lower	< 5

*June 2012 Current Price Index, Labor Bureau, Ministry of Labor, Government of India. Linking factors between new series and old series. Available from: http://labourbureau.nic.in/indexes.htm.

Index

W

Y

Z